Feature Extraction by Neurons and Behavior

edited by
Gerhard Werner

The MIT Press
Massachusetts Institute of Technology
Cambridge, Massachusetts

FEATURE EXTRACTION BY NEURONS AND BEHAVIOR

Introduction

GERHARD WERNER

As AN ALTERNATIVE to the exhaustive specification of sensory input by neural activity in afferent pathways, coding schemes that reduce redundancy in sensory stimuli have attracted attention since the mid-1950s (Attneave, 1954; Barlow, 1959). The underlying notion was that evolutionary adaptation of the organisms to certain types of redundancies, which are always present in the environment, would have occurred. The guiding principle in these considerations was Shannon's concept of "optimal codes," which match the statistical structure of regularities in the available repertoire of messages.

As far as it was known at that time, there were only two mechanisms available to the nervous system to reduce redundancy of information in the stimulus. These were, in the temporal domain, mechanisms specifically sensitive to onset and cessation of a stimulus; and in the spatial domain, lateral inhibition. The potential significance of such redundancy reducing codes consists of economy in signal transmission, because these codes exploit lawful regularities in the stimulus source. For instance, the duration of a stationary stimulus is uniquely defined by the moments of its beginning and end, and thus there is no need for generating neuronal impulses in the interval between these points in time.

The concept of the "stimulus feature" can be considered a generalization of this principle. This concept becomes applicable whenever a neuronal discharge signals with relatively high selectivity the occurrence of an input state that contains in its specifications the concomitant occurrence of certain regularities in the stimulus space, in addition to being specific for a certain place on the receptor sheet and stimulus modality. For instance, because matter is cohesive, objects can be fully characterized in terms of their boundaries; hence, boundaries (that is, edges, corners, and angles) become the "features" in terms of which the spatial layout of a stimulus object can be unambiguously represented.

Such features may be purely of a spatial nature, consisting of stationary contours or patterns, or they may combine spatial with temporal information in the form of a stimulus motion. The economy consists, then, of limiting the characterization of a shape to the signaling of its boundaries, or of emphasizing change over stationarity.

Carried to its logical consequence, this principle implies that the central nervous system takes the information available in the proximal stimulus on receptor sheets out of its original context and imposes a classification into disjunctive entities. The general principle appears to be that the number of neurons available to signal stimulus information increases with progression along the afferent pathway but that any given neuron is less frequently activated as the constraints of its stimulus feature become more severe (Barlow, 1969).

The neurophysiological reality of feature detection is by now amply substantiated; however, it also raises many problems. This is most aptly captured in the concluding sentence of a paper by Hubel and Wiesel (1968):

Specialized as the cells of area 17 are, compared with rods and cones, they must, nevertheless, still represent a very elementary stage in handling complex forms, occupied as they are with a relatively simple region-by-region analysis of retinal contours. How this information is used at later stages in the visual path is far from clear and represents one of the most tantalizing problems for the future.

These problems range from clarifying in neurophysiological experiments the synaptic mechanisms enabling feature detection to establishing the perceptual relevance of feature-sensitive neurons by psychological means.

This latter issue comes into sharper focus if we ask the question which place and what role feature-signaling neurons in the nervous system could play in a mechanistic account of behavioral and perceptual functions and in a psychological theory of information processing. To illustrate contrasting possibilities of their involvement, we may consider features as a hierarchy of elements in terms of which entire scenes of sensory input are analyzed and described (Barlow, Narasimhan, and Rosenfeld, 1972); alternatively, we may consider that feature elements stand at the interface between perception and action, in the sense that they trigger or "release" behavioral acts in an automatalike fashion.

Irrespective of our theoretical biases and inclinations, these are fundamental problems in trying to bring behavioral performance into register with current neurophysiological concepts. To some extent, at least, these problems are a consequence of the manner in which neurophysiological experiments characterize and identify stimulus feature-sensitive neurons, namely, by observing electrical activity in individual neurons, one at a time. The correlated perceptual activity, on the other hand, involves global activity in complex neural systems.

These comments are intended to underscore some of the principal issues to which the following papers in this part are addressed.

REFERENCES

Attneave, F., 1954. Informational aspects of visual perception. *Psychol. Rev.* 61:183–193.

Barlow, H. B., 1959. Sensory mechanisms, the reduction of redundancy and intelligence. Symposium on the mechanization of thought processes at the National Physical Laboratory, London. H.M. Stationery Office, Symp. No. 10, 535–539.

Barlow, H. B., 1969. Trigger features, adaptation and economy of impulses. In *Information Processing in the Nervous System*, K. N. Leibovic, ed. Berlin: Springer-Verlag.

Barlow, H. B., R. Narasimhan, and A. Rosenfeld, 1972. Visual pattern analysis in machines and animals. *Science* 177: 567–575.

Hubel, D. H., and T. N. Wiesel, 1968. Receptive fields and functional architecture of monkey striate cortex. *J. Physiol.* (*London*) 195:215–243.

9 The Transmission of Spatial Information through the Visual System

FERGUS W. CAMPBELL

ABSTRACT The contrast threshold of grating patterns with a variety of wave forms is examined. The thresholds, over a wide range of spatial frequency, can be accounted for by the simple application of Fourier theory. It is suggested that there may be in the visual system channels tuned to spatial frequency because it has been shown neurophysiologically, in the cat and monkey, that the neurons discovered in the cortex by Hubel and Wiesel are indeed sharply tuned to spatial frequency as well as orientation. The analogy of this mechanism with the one present in the auditory system for pitch transmission has led to many psychophysical experiments to test how useful this paradigm is in accounting for established visual phenomena and for predicting the visibility of other test patterns.

THE THEOREM OF Fourier (1768–1830) enabled Helmholtz (1821–1894) to make his contribution to our understanding of the physical nature of music and to the first scientific attempt to unravel the physiology of hearing. We know from his biographer, Koenigsberger (1965), that Helmholtz "had for years gone to bed and got up again with Fourier's series in his mind," and it is therefore surprising that he did not apply with equal success Fourier's technique to optics and to the physiology of the eye.

Helmholtz came very near to considering it, for Koenigsberger (1965) reports that Helmholtz thought that "the eye has no harmony in the same sense as the ear; it has no music." In making this comparison between the eye and the ear, Helmholtz was contrasting color vision with that of harmony; for the ear can analyze a compound sound into its frequency components while the eye cannot resolve a compound color into its component spectral wavelengths. Half a century had to pass before the first step was taken by Duffieux (1946) to apply Fourier theory to physical optics. It could well have been done by Helmholtz.

I hope to show you that harmony is certainly present in the visual sense, but it is in the domain of space and not of color.

We know from experience that as an object recedes from us it becomes increasingly difficult to perceive its details until, at a sufficiently great distance, the object itself disappears from view. Alice, in *Through the Looking-Glass*, once remarked "I see nobody on the road," and the White King replied in a fretful tone "I only wish I had such eyes, to be able to see nobody and at that distance too."

Many factors have been put forward to account for this everyday experience. For example, the limits of visual acuity may be restricted by the optical properties of the eye, or by the dimensions of the foveal mosaic of cones, or by the rate at which light quanta are captured by individual photoreceptors (Rose, 1970) or even by limitations within the visual nervous system itself. In order to solve this problem in an analytical manner, it is necessary to measure the transmission of spatial signals through each part of the system. To do this it is essential to choose an input signal that produces a fairly simple output signal. We have chosen to use the mathematically simplest spatial signal of all—a grating whose luminance varies sinusoidally along one axis (see Campbell, 1968, and Figure 1 for illustration). This is the homologue of a pure tone in the auditory system.

We are going to consider the following elements to be in cascade and investigate the transmission properties of each section in turn; object → image → ganglion cell → geniculate fiber → visual cortex neuron → psychophysics → ?

This approach for investigating the transmission of information through a system is really borrowed from electrical engineering where the attenuation and amplification of temporal signals is important. Hopkins (1962), O'Neill (1963), and Linfoot (1964) have already successfully developed Fourier theory to a point where many optical systems can be precisely and analytically described in this manner.

Arnulf and Dupuy (1960) and Westheimer (1960) were the first to realize the power of this approach in visual optics and they used a technique invented earlier by Le Grand (1937). They passed coherent beams of light into the eye and set up a sinusoidal interference grating on the retina using the principle of Thomas Young (Young, 1800). This ingenious technique bypasses the defects that might arise from aberrations in the optical components of

FERGUS W. CAMPBELL The Physiological Laboratory, Cambridge, England

FIGURE 1 The grating has a sinusoidal wave form of constant spatial frequency. Its contrast is changing logarithmically from about 0.4 to about 0.004. Due to nonlinearities in the photographic process, the wave form is not sinusoidal at high contrast levels. The reader should observe the grating from different distances and note the change in the threshold contrast with spatial frequency.

the eye, and it permitted them to establish the resolving power of the retina, coupled to the brain, in isolation from the dioptrics. Unfortunately, the complete success of this experiment depends upon having a monochromatic source with a high degree of coherence and also high luminance.

Such a source became available when the neon-helium laser was invented. Using it, Campbell and Green (1965) were able to show that the fundal image formed by a well-focused eye, with a normal-sized pupil, was surprisingly good and that most of the loss of contrast in the perception of fine gratings was due to the properties of the retina and/or brain. The transmission properties of the dioptrics have also been measured directly using an objective method (Campbell and Gubisch, 1966) and the results obtained by these two fundamentally different methods agree well.

The results of change of pupil size as well as those of focus have been investigated (Green and Campbell, 1965). Green (1967) has demonstrated the effects of off-axis aberrations and Campbell and Gubisch (1967) have shown the effect of the chromatic aberration present in the eye on the contrast sensitivity function.

All of these experiments indicate that the quality of the retinal image in an emmetrope is very good. Thus at high light levels, the resolution is limited mainly by the properties of the retina and/or brain. At low light levels, the main limit is the number of photons being captured per cone per integration time (about 1/10 sec).

These approaches have so far been useful in finding out the nature of the fundal image (Gubisch, 1967); but can these be used to further our understanding of how spatial signals are transmitted and transformed by the nervous system itself?

The first convenient level at which spatial signals can be detected is at the ganglion cells that transmit the signals from the retina to the geniculate body. Enroth-Cugell and Robson (1966), using sinusoidal gratings generated on the face of an oscilloscope, have studied the response of these cells in the cat. In this animal, the direction of movement of a grating is unimportant as the cells respond equally to movement in all directions. They found one class of cells that responded in a linear manner to their stimuli. A finding, which may be of great significance, was that each cell responded only over a limited range of spatial frequency. The properties of these linear ganglion cells have been further studied by Cleland, Dubin, and Levick (1971).

The fibers from the geniculate body terminate in the striate visual cortex, and their activity can readily be monitored by microelectrodes (Hubel, 1957). Cooper and Robson (1968) and Campbell, Cooper, and Enroth-Cugell (1969) find that at this level the geniculate units again respond only to limited bands of spatial frequency. Like the ganglion cells, the geniculate units respond to movement in all directions.

However, the cells in the striate visual cortex behave quite differently, as has been most elegantly shown by Hubel and Wiesel (1959, 1962, and 1965), in the cat and also in the monkey (Hubel and Wiesel, 1968). Here the cells are very sensitive to the orientation of an edge or bar when it is moved across the receptive field. Using grating patterns Campbell, Cleland, Cooper, and Enroth-Cugell (1968) have measured quantitatively this selectivity to orientation in the cat. These orientationally selective cells will, of course, also respond to a grating providing it is moved at the optimum orientation. These cortical cells also respond to only limited bands of spatial frequencies, each cell responding to a different range in the spectrum of spatial frequencies (Cooper and Robson, 1968; Campbell, Cooper, and Enroth-Cugell, 1969). There is some preliminary evidence (Campbell, Cooper, Robson, and Sachs, 1969) that neurons in the cortex of the monkey are similarly organized.

These neurophysiological findings in the cat and monkey suggest that two important properties of an image have been coded. First, the information about orientation of an edge, bar, or grating is extracted. Second, the spatial frequency content of the image is also extracted.

This organization is strikingly similar to that found in the auditory system where units are found that respond to pure-tone bursts over a limited range of pitch (Kiang, 1966), rather like the neurons of the visual cortex that respond over a limited range of spatial frequency. Again, in the auditory cortex neurons are found that only respond to either a rise or a fall of pitch (Whitfield and Evans, 1965); indeed, because of their resemblance to the visual cortical cells, they have been called "directional cells" (Whitfield, 1967).

Is there any evidence that the visual system of man is similarly organized? If such organization can be demonstrated, it will greatly strengthen the argument that these neurophysiological findings are directly relevant properties of the mechanism by which we perceive, and possibly recognize, objects.

Campbell and Kulikowski (1966) attempted to show that man has channels sensitive to the orientation of a grating by measuring psychophysically the threshold of a test grating in the presence of a high-contrast masking grating. They changed the orientation of the masking grating relative to the test grating and found that maximum masking occurred when the two gratings had the same orientation and that no masking occurred when the masking grating was at right angles to the test grating. For intermediate angles, the masking effect decreased exponentially; the masking effect was reduced by half when the angle between the gratings was only 12° to 15°. Man seems to have a slightly higher orientational selectivity than the cat (Campbell, Cleland, Cooper, and Enroth-Cugell, 1968) and may resemble more closely the monkey (Hubel and Wiesel, 1968) where the angular selectivity was found to be higher than that of the cat. Thus, as far as orientation performance is concerned, there is a striking agreement between the neurophysiology and the psychophysics.

Can we show that man also has channels selectively sensitive to spatial frequency? In a preliminary note, Campbell and Robson (1964) suggested that Fourier theory might be applied to the psychophysics of spatial vision. In their main paper (Campbell and Robson, 1968), they measured the contrast threshold for a number of gratings each with a different wave form. They found that the threshold is determined by the amplitude of the fundamental Fourier component in the grating and that the higher harmonics do not contribute to the threshold, providing they are below their own threshold. In like manner, a square-wave grating can be distinguished from a sinusoidal-wave grating when the contrast is sufficiently high for the third harmonic to be detected in the presence of the fundamental. Their findings led them to suggest that there must be a number of channels in the human visual system each tuned to different spatial frequencies. They thought that the effective bandwidth of each channel is probably not greater than about one octave of spatial frequency.

In 1966, Campbell and Kulikowski used the technique of masking a low-contrast test grating with a high-contrast grating of the same orientation and spatial frequency. In undertaking these experiments they found that it was necessary to have the two gratings of the same spatial frequency or the masking effect was much less. Gilinsky (1967, 1968) developed this masking method further by adapting for some time to a grating of a given frequency and then subsequently inspecting the test grating that was at a different orientation. Using her adaptation method, Pantle and Sekuler (1968) studied the influence of gratings with the same orientation but with different spatial frequencies on each other. They summarize their findings as: "These conclusions are similar to those reached by Campbell and Robson (1968) from a Fourier analysis of the visibility of gratings of different spatial frequencies and wave forms."

Unfortunately, Pantle and Sekuler (1968) used square-wave gratings to produce their adaptation effects, and this complicates the interpretation of their data, for the higher Fourier components in their gratings also influenced the results. By using sinusoidal gratings covering a wide range of spatial frequency, Blakemore and Campbell (1969) were able to measure accurately the bandwidth of each channel and also to demonstrate that there were many channels. In these experiments the subject adapted to a given frequency, and the loss in contrast sensitivity was measured at, and on either side of, that frequency, (open circles, and right-hand and upper scale of Figure 2). The "bandwidth" of the adaptation effect is about ±1 octave. Also, the response of a single neuron from the cortex of the cat is plotted in this figure (closed circles, and left-hand and lower scale). The adaptation technique of Blakemore and Campbell shows that there are channels tuned to spatial frequencies ranging from 3 c/deg up to the upper limit of resolution at about 48 c/deg.

Blakemore and Campbell (1969) noticed that, if a subject adapted to a square-wave grating, the threshold for detecting both the fundamental and the third harmonic was elevated. Tolhurst (1972b) has examined this phenomenon more quantitatively by adapting to both square waves and also the fundamental with its third harmonic. He finds that, for high levels of adapting contrast, the presence of more than one grating reduces the

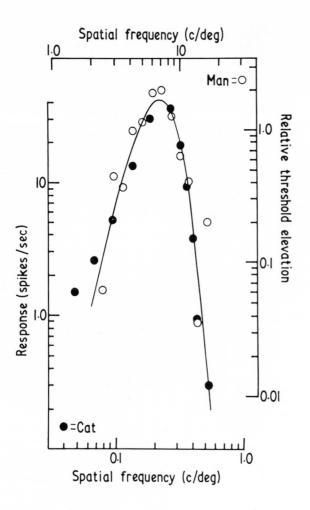

FIGURE 2　The closed circles (●) are the responses (spikes/sec) from an orientational cortical neuron from a cat. The sinusoidal grating stimulus had a contrast of 0.5 and was drifting in the preferred direction so that one bar of the grating passed the receptive field each second (Results supplied by J. G. Robson and G. F. Cooper, the Physiological Laboratory, Cambridge).

The open circles (○) are the relative threshold elevations in man produced by adapting to a sinusoidal grating of contrast 0.7 and spatial frequency 7 c/deg (Blakemore and Campbell, 1969).

To compare the response of this particular cat neuron with the psychophysical adaptation, the data has been superimposed to obtain the best fit by eye and the appropriate scales attached. It must be emphasized that there is a range of cortical neurons each responding maximally to a different spatial frequency (Campbell, Cooper, and Enroth-Cugell, 1969; Campbell, Cooper, Robson, and Sachs, 1969). Likewise, in the human, adaptation to different spatial frequencies reveals a comparable range of tuned channels (Blakemore and Campbell, 1969).

The curve through the results is

$$s = (e^{-f^2} - e^{-(2f)^2})^3$$

where s = contrast sensitivity and f = spatial frequency.

adaptation effect. He postulates that there is mutual inhibition between the fundamental and its third harmonic at these suprathreshold contrast levels; at or near threshold, there is no such reciprocal inhibition.

Sharpe (1972) has studied the fading of retinal capillaries and arterioles when they are stabilized on the retina. He finds that the fading is influenced not only by the orientation of a given capillary but also by its spatial frequency or size. His results can be explained in terms of adaptation (Blakemore and Campbell, 1969) of spatial frequency and orientation channels.

The basic idea that there might be, in vision, channels tuned to spatial frequency has been taken up in audition, and adaptation to frequency modulated tones has been discovered (Kay and Matthews, 1971, 1972).

Campbell and Maffei (1970) and Maffei and Campbell (1970) have developed a technique for using the evoked potential recorded from the visual area of the scalp to obtain an objective measure for the existence of these channels. In this manner, the response of the observer is not required, for thresholds can be determined objectively. They have effectively removed the psycho from psychophysics. They confirm, at the level where the evoked potential arises, that there is a mechanism generating an electrical signal that is selectively sensitive to spatial frequency and orientation, just as has been shown in the previous single neuron and psychophysical studies.

Campbell and Kulikowski (1972) have shown that this evoked potential technique predicts objectively the 50% probability of seeing in the contrast domain.

Blakemore, Nachmias, and Sutton (1970) have shown that if one adapts to a grating of a slightly lower or higher frequency, the lower frequency appears of even lower frequency; conversely the higher frequency appears to be of even higher frequency (Figure 3). This supports the original suggestion by Blakemore and Campbell (1969) that these channels, selective to spatial frequency, may be used for coding the sizes of objects. Sachs, Nachmias, and Robson (1971) have shown psychophysically that each channel is independent from its neighbor by testing the effect on the threshold of mixing two different spatial frequencies. Even when the frequencies are quite close in period, they only add according to the laws of probability summation; in other words the channels are functionally separate. An implication from their measurements is that the bandwidth of the channels being measured in their way is very much narrower than ± 1 octave.

Graham and Nachmias (1971) measured contrast thresholds for gratings containing two superimposed sinusoidal components; the frequency of one component was always three times that of the other, but the phase between the components could be varied so that the sum

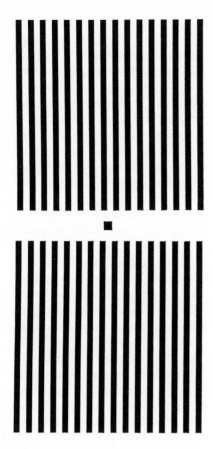 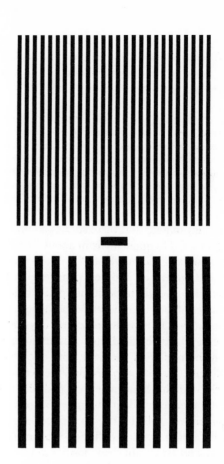

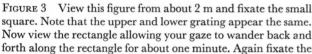

FIGURE 3 View this figure from about 2 m and fixate the small square. Note that the upper and lower grating appear the same. Now view the rectangle allowing your gaze to wander back and forth along the rectangle for about one minute. Again fixate the square and note the change in the appearance of the gratings which were previously identical. (From Blakemore and Sutton, 1969.)

of their contrasts took on several values. Two models of pattern vision were then tested: (1) a single-channel model in which pattern vision is a function of a single neural network and (2) a multiple-channel model in which the stimulus information is processed by many channels, each selectively sensitive to a narrow range of spatial frequencies. Their clear-cut results support the multiple-channel and convincingly reject the single-channel model.

Graham (1972) went on to study the sensitivity of these channels for patterns at low mean luminance or high drift rate. She found that the channels did not behave in the way expected from retinal ganglion cell neurophysiology. Instead, the channels remained selectively sensitive to narrow ranges of spatial frequency even when the luminance was low and the drift rate was high—conditions that tend to affect the inhibitory surround of ganglion cells.

A long-lasting color aftereffect, specific to edge orien-

tation was first demonstrated by McCollough (1965). She found that the effect could be built up by viewing a vertical grating of black stripes upon one color that alternated with a horizontal grating on another color. Complementary colored aftereffects were seen on test gratings of black and white stripes, with the provision that the retinal orientation was similar to the adapting gratings. Stromeyer (1972) has found that the McCollough effect is spatial frequency specific; that is, the effect gets weaker the greater the difference in spatial frequency between the adapting and test frequency. He also found that the same orientation could be used and the color effects be generated by adapting at two different spatial frequencies. The aftereffects could then be varied by the apparent frequency shift (Blakemore and Sutton, 1969); however, the interocular transfer of the frequency shift had no effect on the color aftereffect.

Using this wide range of experimental approaches in the cat, monkey, and man, it has been possible to show that the original paradigm of Campbell and Robson (1964, 1968) is productive in the sense that it has suggested a number of novel experiments, each of which confirmed their original suggestion:

Thus a picture emerges of functionally separate mechanisms in the visual nervous system each responding maximally at some particular spatial frequency and hardly at all at spatial frequencies differing by a factor of two. The frequency selectivity of these mechanisms must be determined by integrative processes in the nervous system and they appear to a first approximation at least, to operate linearly (Campbell and Robson, 1968).

It is important to note that these studies confine themselves to high spatial frequencies from about 1 to 50 c/deg in the human and from about 0.1 to 5 c/deg in the cat. At lower spatial frequencies another picture emerges. It seems unlikely that we will understand spatial vision until the performance of the visual system at both high and low spatial frequencies is fully understood and integrated.

If we observe a bipartite field whose luminance changes gradually in the middle of the field from one level to a slightly different one (a ramp profile), we see an extra narrow dark, or light, band at either end of the ramp where the luminance gradient changes abruptly. These spurious bands are called after the discoverer, Ernst Mach (Ratliff, 1965). A related illusion was described by Craik (1940) and was published posthumously (Craik, 1966). Here the two half-fields have the same luminance, but a single sawtoothed notch is introduced between the half-fields. This spatial transient makes the half-fields appear unequally bright. Cornsweet (1970) enhanced the illusion by using adjacent positive and negative sawtoothed luminance notches (Brindley, 1970, Fig. 6.3). The remarkable finding about the Craik-Cornsweet illusion is that having disturbed the uniform luminance by this localized spatial transient the visual system continues to be misled about the luminance of the field for a considerable distance away from the transient.

Campbell, Howell, and Robson (1971) have developed another way of showing this effect. A grating pattern with uniform light and dark bars is generated on the face of an oscilloscope. The spatial frequency of the grating must be less than 1 c/deg and the contrast must not be too high. As expected, the grating looks as if it had a square-wave distribution of luminance. Now we subtract from the square wave its fundamental Fourier component, leaving intact all the higher components—the third, fifth, and higher odd harmonics. Surprisingly, the pattern still looks as though it had a square wave luminance distribution. It seems that at these low spatial frequencies it is the higher harmonics alone that generate the square wave appearance of the grating. The missing luminance due to the absent fundamental has been "filled in."

Now consider what would be seen if we were to remove the higher harmonics of the square wave grating leaving only the fundamental spatial frequency. When this is done we observe that the screen is of uniform luminance; the low frequency fundamental is not perceived at all. This failure to see the fundamental is not unexpected in view of the well-known increase in the contrast threshold that occurs for spatial frequencies less than 3 c/deg (Robson, 1966; Campbell and Robson, 1968). When this illusion is considered in terms of harmonic analysis, it is no longer surprising that removing the fundamental from a square wave does not appreciably change its appearance, for the fundamental on its own is not detectable.

If we repeat the observations at higher spatial frequencies, we do notice the absence of the fundamental, presumably because the fundamental is not being attenuated relative to the higher harmonics.

It could be argued that there is another type of neuron with odd symmetry in its line-weighting function. These neurons may signal the presence of a transient of contrast, that is, an edge (Tolhurst, 1972a).

The availability of lasers and high-capacity digital computers has made it feasible to apply spatial filtering techniques to the problem of picture analyses. A well-illustrated introduction to these techniques has been prepared by Andrews (1972), and Chapter 10 of Lipson (1972) is very lucid. The practical problems that arise in making an object recognition device are of direct relevance to solving the problem of how we recognize familiar objects in complex scenes. Conversely, pattern recognition engineers are very interested in the visual system, for here is a device that actually works surprisingly well. Ginsburg (1971) has based his approach on the Kabrisky model of the visual system. He has shown that we only require quite a narrow range of low spatial frequency information to recognize many objects. Campbell, Carpenter, and Switkes (1971) are developing methods for filtering scenes using the transmission characteristics of single, and combinations of, neurons.

Using gratings with a sinusoidal luminance profile Campbell and Howell (1972) have been able to demonstrate monocular rivalry. If two gratings with sinusoidal luminance profiles are projected upon a white screen and if they are at right angles to each other, the appearance of the gratings changes continuously. If the gratings are of different color, the effect is seen even more dramatically. Say the gratings are red and green and their intensities are matched so that yellow is perceived where they cross, one then observes that sometimes the red grating is seen on its own and at other times only the green grating is observed. There are periods when both gratings are seen together, but there are never periods when both disappear. In other words, the gratings are seen to alternate.

If the two gratings have the same orientation, and the red bars of one are superimposed on the green bars of the other, then a yellow and black grating is observed, just as one would expect from the rules of color mixing. If the gratings are interdigitated by putting them out-of-phase by 180°, a red-green grating is perceived; no yellow is observed between the red and green sections. This is surprising, for in this region of the sinusoidal distribution the amounts of red and green are such that they previously produced yellow.

With the interdigitated grating, there is no alternation; the appearance is quite stable and unified. Thus, the alternation observed when the gratings were crossed cannot be due to factors such as chromatic aberration of fluctuations of accommodation. Likewise, the alternations cannot be caused by chromatic stereopsis or changes in convergence, for the alternations are observed when one eye is covered. It is not necessary to fixate on any part of the grating, and the pattern of eye movement does not significantly affect the alternation.

The interesting question arises, what is the angle required between the two gratings to produce alternation? If the phenomenon had some simple physical explanation, we might expect the rate of the alternations to increase gradually from 0° to 90°, say as a sine function. It is easy to demonstrate that this is not so; the gratings do not begin to alternate until they are tilted relative to each other by about 15–20°. This orientational selectivity is similar to that found psychophysically by Campbell and Kulikowski (1966) and shown in the cortical neurons of the cat (Campbell, Cleland, Cooper, and Enroth-Cugell, 1968).

The alternations that occur with crossed sinusoidal gratings do not depend upon the colors used, and the phenomenon can be demonstrated with either widely separated wavelengths, such as blue and red, or closely spaced colors such as yellow and yellow-green. While the effect is very dramatic when the gratings differ in color, color difference is not essential to obtain the alternation. It will work if the two gratings are the same color or are white.

If gratings with a square-wave luminance profile are used, the rate of alternation is slower. In the case of sinusoidal gratings, one grating can disappear completely, but with square-wave gratings, complete disappearance does not occur; only a weak attenuation of apparent contrast is observed.

Similar alternations occur with two crossed bars, with the provision that the bars are sufficiently blurred to remove the higher spatial frequencies in the image of the cross. This makes a useful and simple lecture-room demonstration of the orientational selectivity of the visual system discovered by Hubel and Wiesel in 1959.

One could explain this monocular rivalry on the assumption that orientations and spatial frequencies are processed in independent channels that are highly selective ($\pm 15°$ and ± 1 octave). For some unknown reason, first one channel dominates and then the other. It would be interesting to see if this alternation occurs in individual neurons in the cat or monkey.

Why has the experimental application of elementary Fourier theory so far worked so well? Its strict application demands that the system being studied be linear; that is, that the principle of superposition holds. We have used the theory only because it is the queen of all description and also because it is easy to explain the results and their implications to a wide public. It does not follow that it is the best one, or even ultimately the correct one. Since the visual system has neurons tuned to each orientation, it seems empirically sensible to use a one-dimensional function for studying these later stages of signal transmission.

It is true that the fact that a threshold exists means that there is indeed a nonlinearity. However, for threshold measurements this nonlinearity is easy to handle mathematically. The visual system is grossly nonlinear when the dynamics of dark and light adaptation are involved. We have always eschewed this complication by restricting our studies to the performance of the eye at one mean light level. Likewise, the visual system is nonlinear if it is overloaded with very high contrast levels. We have confined ourselves to levels of contrast less than 0.7, which covers almost all of the range used in normal sight, providing one does not look directly at light sources or subject the eye to glare. The contrast of the print that you are now reading is 0.7.

It would be rather disappointing if this internal consistency for the prediction of thresholds for different types of objects was restricted to repetitive patterns, such as gratings, and not to other more interesting and realistic objects such as surround us in daily life. Campbell, Carpenter, and Levinson (1969) have attempted to predict the thresholds of thin lines and bars from the contrast sensitivity function. They find that it is possible to do this, again using a linear theory (Fourier).

Sullivan, Georgeson, and Oatley (1972) have studied the effect of adapting to gratings on the subsequent threshold for bars of different width. They find that bar width and spatial frequency are not equivalent and that there is no evidence for width selective channels. Bars seem to be detected when their frequency components most easily detected by the visual system (near 5 c/deg) rise above their independent thresholds.

Carter and Henning (1971) have designed some experiments to test whether the behavior of the eye can be considered as similar to the behavior of Helmholtz's model of the ear. Their experiments are analogous to some auditory experiments of Wightman and Leshowitz (1970) and Leshowitz and Wightman (1971). The detectibility of sinusoidal gratings comprised of either one or many cycles was measured in veiling luminances, the spatial frequencies of which were either narrow or broad-band. In narrow-band noise, the single-cycle grating was detected with approximately 0.6 log units less contrast than the many-cycle grating. On the other hand, when both broad-band and narrow-band noise were present, there was no measureable difference in the detectability of the two types of grating. Carter and Henning (1971) consider critically a number of detection models to account for their results and conclude

In any case, it is clear that the concept of the energy density spectrum of the object grating, together with the Campbell and Robson (1968) hypothesis that the visual system analyses spatial frequencies in separate bands, leads to qualitatively predictable results.

I may not have convinced you that the visual system really does have harmony, but you may now agree that it will be in the domain of spatial frequency and contrast, and not color, where we will appreciate the harmony of which Helmholtz might well have dreamed. Today it would be difficult to imagine our concepts of sound, music, and audition if Fourier had not gifted Helmholtz with this approach. In audition it has brought some order out of chaos (Helmholtz, 1877), although much remains to be understood. The history of the application of the Fourier series in vision lies in the future. It may be short, it may be long; at least it should be interesting.

NOTES ADDED IN PROOF Maffei and Fiorentini (1972) showed that the information about the amplitude and phase of two sinusoidal stimuli, presented separately to the two eyes, can be synthesized by the visual system. Results indicate that this process of synthesis can be described in terms of Fourier theory, at least for relatively low contrast, and nervous operators exist that are able to rebuild the image from its sinusoidal components. (L. Maffei, and A. Fiorentini, 1972, *Nature* 240:479–481.) Bodis-Wollner (1972) measured the contrast sensitivity function on two patients with neurological disorders in the visual cortex and finds that, although visual acuity is only slightly decreased, they have markedly decreased contrast sensitivity at all spatial frequencies particularly at intermediate and high spatial frequencies. He coins the term visuogram for this clinical method. (I. Bodis-Wollner, 1972, *Science* 178:769–771.)

REFERENCES

ANDREWS, H. C., 1972. Digital computers and image processing. *Endeavour* 31 (113): 88–94.

ARNULF, A., and O. DUPUY, 1960. La transmission des contrastes par le système optique de l'oeil et les seuils des contrastes rétiniens. *Compt. Rend. Acad. Sci.* 250: 2727–2759.

BLAKEMORE, C., and F. W. CAMPBELL, 1969. On the existence in the human visual system of neurons selectively sensitive to the orientation and size of retinal images. *J. Physiol.* (*London*) 203:237–260.

BLAKEMORE, C., J. NACHMIAS, and P. SUTTON, 1970. The perceived spatial frequency shift: Evidence for frequency selective neurons in the human brain. *J. Physiol.* (*London*) 210: 727–750.

BLAKEMORE, C., and P. SUTTON, 1969. Size adaption: The new aftereffect. *Science* 166:245–247.

BRINDLEY, G. S., 1970. *Physiology of the Retina and Visual Pathway*, 2nd ed. London: Edward Arnold (Publishers) Ltd.

CAMPBELL, F. W., 1968. The human eye as an optical filter. *Proc. IEEE* 56:1009.

CAMPBELL, F. W., R. H. S. CARPENTER, and J. Z. LEVINSON, 1969. Visibility of aperiodic patterns compared with that of sinusoidal gratings. *J. Physiol.* (*London*) 204:283–298.

CAMPBELL, F. W., R. H. S. CARPENTER, and E. SWITKES, 1971. Simple scanning devices for computer modelling of visual processes. *J. Physiol.* (*London*) 217:18–19.

CAMPBELL, F. W., B. C. CLELAND, G. F. COOPER, and CHRISTINA ENROTH-CUGELL, 1968. The angular selectivity of visual cortical cells to moving gratings. *J. Physiol.* (*London*) 198: 237–250.

CAMPBELL, F. W., G. F. COOPER, and CHRISTINA ENROTH-CUGELL, 1969. The spatial selectivity of the visual cells of the cat. *J. Physiol.* (*London*) 203:223–235.

CAMPBELL, F. W., G. F. COOPER, J. G. ROBSON, and M. B. SACHS, 1969. The spatial selectivity of visual cells of the cat and the squirrel monkey. *J. Physiol.* (*London*) 204: 120–121.

CAMPBELL, F. W., and D. G. GREEN, 1965. Optical and retinal factors affecting visual resolution. *J. Physiol.* (*London*) 181: 576–593.

CAMPBELL, F. W., and R. W. GUBISCH, 1966. Optical quality of the human eye. *J. Physiol.* (*London*) 186:558–578.

CAMPBELL, F. W., and R. W. GUBISCH, 1967. The effect of chromatic aberration on visual acuity. *J. Physiol.* (*London*) 192:345–359.

CAMPBELL, F. W., and E. R. HOWELL, 1972. Monocular alternation: A method for the investigation of pattern vision. *J. Physiol.* (*London*) 222:19–21.

CAMPBELL, F. W., E. R. HOWELL, and J. G. ROBSON, 1971. The appearance of gratings with and without the fundamental Fourier component. *J. Physiol.* (*London*) 217:17–18.

CAMPBELL, F. W., and J. J. KULIKOWSKI, 1966. Orientational selectivity of the human visual system. *J. Physiol.* (*London*) 187: 437–445.

CAMPBELL, F. W., and J. J. KULIKOWSKI, 1972. The visual evoked potential as a function of contrast of a grating pattern. *J. Physiol.* (*London*) 222:345–356.

CAMPBELL, F. W., and L. MAFFEI, 1970. Electrophysiological evidence for the existence of orientation and size detectors in the human visual system. *J. Physiol.* (*London*) 207:635–652.

CAMPBELL, F. W., J. NACHMIAS, and J. JUKES, 1970. Spatial-frequency discrimination in human vision. *J. Opt. Soc. Am.* 60:555–559.

CAMPBELL, F. W., and J. G. ROBSON, 1964. Application of Fourier analysis to the modulation response of the eye. *J. Opt. Soc. Am.* 54:581.

CAMPBELL, F. W., and J. G. ROBSON, 1968. Application of Fourier analysis to the visibility of gratings. *J. Physiol.* (*London*) 197:551–566.

CARTER, B. E., and G. B. HENNING, 1971. The detection of gratings in narrow-band visual noise. *J. Physiol.* (*London*) 219: 355–365.

CLELAND, B. G., M. W. DUBIN, and W. R. LEVICK, 1971. Sustained and transient neurons in the cat's retina and lateral geniculate nucleus. *J. Physiol. (London)* 217:473–496.

COOPER, G. F., and J. G. ROBSON, 1968. Successive transformations of spatial information in the visual system. Conference on pattern recognition, N.P.L. Inst. of Elec. Eng., London.

CORNSWEET, T. N., 1970. *Visual Perception.* New York and London: Academic Press.

CRAIK, K. J. W., 1940. Visual Adaptation. Ph.D. dissertation, University of Cambridge.

CRAIK, K. J. W., 1966. *The Nature of Psychology*, Sherwood, S. L., ed. Cambridge University Press.

DUFFIEUX, P. M., 1946. L'integrale de Fourier et ses applications a l'optique. Privately printed (Besancon).

ENROTH-CUGELL, CHRISTINA, and J. G. ROBSON, 1966. The contrast sensitivity of retinal ganglion cells of the cat. *J. Physiol. (London)* 187:517–552.

GILINSKY, ALBERTA S., 1967. Masking of contour-detectors in the human visual system. *Psychon. Sci.* 8:395–396.

GILINSKY, ALBERTA S., 1968. Orientation-specific effects of patterns of adapting light on visual acuity. *J. Opt. Soc. Am.* 58:13–18.

GINSBURG, A. P., 1971. Psychological Correlates of a Model of the Human Visual System. Masters thesis, Air Force Institute of Technology, Wright-Patterson AFB, Ohio 45433.

GRAHAM, NORMA, 1972. Spatial frequency channels in the human visual system: Effects of luminance and pattern drift rate. *Vision Res.* 12:53–68.

GRAHAM, N., and J. NACHMIAS, 1971. Detection of grating patterns containing two spatial frequencies: A comparison of single-channel and multiple-channel models. *Vision Res.* 11: 251–259.

GREEN, D. G., 1967. Visual resolution when light enters the eye through different parts of the pupil. *J. Physiol. (London)* 190: 583–593.

GREEN, D. G., and F. W. CAMPBELL, 1965. Effect of focus on the visual response to a sinusoidally modulated spatial stimulus. *J. Opt. Soc. Am.* 55:1154.

GUBISCH, R. W., 1967. Optical performance of the human eye. *J. Opt. Soc. Am.* 57:407–415.

HELMHOLTZ, H., 1877. *On the Sensations of Tone.* (Reprinted 1954.) New York: Dover Publications.

HOPKINS, H. H., 1962. 21st Thomas Young Oration. The application of frequency response techniques in optics. *Proc. Phys. Soc. (London)* 79:889–919.

HUBEL, D. H., 1957. Tungsten microelectrode for recording from single units. *Science* 125:549–550.

HUBEL, D. H., and T. N. WIESEL, 1959. Receptive fields of single neurons in the cat's striate cortex. *J. Physiol. (London)* 148:574–591.

HUBEL, D. H., and T. N. WIESEL, 1962. Receptive fields, binocular interaction and functional architecture in the cat's visual cortex. *J. Physiol. (London)* 160:106–154.

HUBEL, D. H., and T. N. WIESEL, 1965. Receptive fields and functional architecture in two nonstriate visual areas (18 and 19) of the cat. *J. Neurophysiol.* 28:229–289.

HUBEL, D. H., and T. N. WIESEL, 1968. Receptive fields and functional architecture of monkey striate cortex. *J. Physiol. (London)* 195:215–243.

KAY, R. H., and D. R. MATTHEWS, 1971. Temporal specificity in human auditory conditioning by frequency-modulated tones. *J. Physiol. (London)* 218:104–106.

KAY, R. H., and D. R. MATTHEWS, 1972. On the existence in human auditory pathways of channels selectively tuned to the modulation present in frequency-modulated tones. *J. Physiol. (London)* 225:657–677.

KIANG, N. Y.-S., 1966. *Discharge Patterns of Single Fibers in the Cat's Auditory Nerve.* Cambridge, Mass., MIT Press.

KOENIGSBERGER, L., 1965. *Hermann von Helmholtz.* New York: Dover Publications.

LE GRAND, Y., 1937. La formation des images retiniennes. Sur un mode de vision éliminant les défauts optiques de l'oeil. Paris: 2e Reunion de l'Institute d'Optique.

LESHOWITZ, B., and F. L. WIGHTMAN, 1971. On-frequency tonal masking. *J. Acoust. Soc. Am.* 49:1180–1190.

LINFOOT, E. H., 1964. *Fourier Methods for Optical Image Evaluation.* London and New York: The Focal Press.

LIPSON, H., 1972. *Optical Transforms.* New York and London: Academic Press.

McCOLLOUGH, C., 1965. Color adaptation of edge-detectors in the human visual system. *Science* 149:1115–1116.

MAFFEI, L., and F. W. CAMPBELL, 1970. Neurophysiological localization of the vertical and horizontal visual coordinates in man. *Science* 167:386–387.

MITCHELL, D. E., R. D. FREEMAN, and G. WESTHEIMER, 1967. Effect of orientation on the modulation sensitivity for interference fringes on the retina. *J. Opt. Soc. Am.* 57:246–249.

O'NEILL, E. L., 1963. *Introduction to Statistical Optics.* Reading, Mass.: Addison-Wesley Publishing Company.

PANTLE, A., and R. SEKULER, 1968. Size-detecting mechanisms in human vision. *Science* 162:1146–1148.

RATLIFF, F., 1965. Mach Bands: Quantitative studies on neural networks in the retina, 1st ed. San Francisco: Holden-Day, 37–169.

ROBSON, J. G., 1966. Spatial and temporal contrast-sensitivity functions of the visual system. *J. Soc. Opt. Am.* 56:1141–1142.

ROSE, A., 1970. Quantum limitations to vision at low light levels. *Image Tech.* 12:13–31.

SACHS, M. B., J. NACHMIAS, and J. G. ROBSON, 1971. Spatial-frequency channels in human vision. *J. Opt. Soc. Am.* 61: 1176–1186.

SHARPE, C. R., 1972. The visibility and fading of thin lines visualized by their controlled movement across the retina. *J. Physiol. (London)* 222:113–134.

STROMEYER, C. F., 1972. Edge-contingent color after effects: spatial frequency specificity. *Vision Res.* 12:717–733.

SULLIVAN, G. D., M. A. GEORGESON, and K. OATLEY, 1972. Channels for spatial frequency selection and the detection of single bars by the human visual system. *Vision Res.* 12:383–394.

TOLHURST, D. J., 1972a. On the possible existence of edge detector neurons in the human visual system. *Vision Res.* 12: 797–804.

TOLHURST, D. J., 1972b. Adaptation to square-wave gratings: inhibition between spatial frequency channels in the human visual system. *J. Physiol. (London)* 226:231–248.

WESTHEIMER, G., 1960. Modulation thresholds for sinusoidal light distributions on the retina. *J. Physiol. (London)* 152: 67–74.

WHITFIELD, I. C., 1967. *The Auditory Pathway.* London: Edward Arnold Ltd.

WHITFIELD, I. C., and E. F. EVANS, 1965. Responses of auditory cortical neurons to stimuli of changing frequency. *J. Neurophysiol.* 28:655–672.

WIGHTMAN, F. L., and B. LESHOWITZ, 1970. Off-frequency tonal masking. *J. Acoust. Soc. Am.* 47A:107.

YOUNG, T., 1800. Outlines of experiments and enquiries respecting sound and light. *Phil. Trans.* 106–150.

10 Developmental Factors in the Formation of Feature Extracting Neurons

COLIN BLAKEMORE

ABSTRACT The final organization of pattern detecting neurons in the visual cortex of a cat is fundamentally determined by the kitten's early visual experience. Exposure, for as little as 1 hour or less, to vertical or horizontal stripes causes virtually every cortical neuron to adopt the experienced orientation as its preferred stimulus. This drastic modification by the environment has a distinct critical period from about 3 weeks to about 14 weeks. Prolonged exposure in an older kitten or an adult has no such effect. This mechanism may be adaptive, the feature-detecting apparatus of the visual system being optimally matched to the animal's visual environment.

Features : Universal or specific?

WHAT COULD BE more compelling than the idea of sensory systems matched precisely to their different sensory worlds? Of course, Johannes Müller (1842) realized that the receptors themselves are specialized to transduce particular forms of energy; but what of the patterns or combinations of stimuli within each modality, which we call *features*? Does a sensory system take an elementary, reductionist approach, treating its input entirely in the simplest possible terms (point-by-point analysis of light on the retina or tone-by-tone analysis of sound in the cochlea, for instance)? Or does it actively search out these complicated patterns of stimuli and disregard rare or meaningless inputs?

We now think that there is, at least within the visual system, a limited repertoire of specific, feature-extracting neurons that the animal uses to deal with its visual world. These neurons work on the signals from the receptors and detect specific spatiotemporal patterns that represent particularly important forms of stimuli. The frog's retina has its bug detectors, edge detectors, and dimming detectors (Lettvin, Maturana, McCulloch, and Pitts, 1959); the rabbit has direction-selective, orientation-selective, and uniformity-detecting ganglion cells in its retina (Barlow and Hill, 1963; Levick, 1967); cats and monkeys, in the visual cortex, have orientation-detecting neurons, which are also sensitive to the stereoscopic dis-

COLIN BLAKEMORE   The Physiological Laboratory, University of Cambridge, Cambridge, England

tance of the stimulus (Hubel and Wiesel, 1962, 1970a; Barlow, Blakemore, and Pettigrew, 1967). In fact every species whose visual pathway has been probed with microelectrodes has been found to possess a limited number of classes of neuron, each sensitive to a particular combination of elementary sensory events, which one could call a feature.

An examination of the results of these experiments shows that there seem to be two kinds of detector neurons:

1. *Universal feature detectors.* These are classes of cell that are found in almost all visual systems, and it seems reasonable to assume that the features they detect are fundamental. These include *temporal transients* (most detector neurons only respond at the beginning or the end of a sudden stimulus); *spatial transients* or *edges* (the process of lateral inhibition in the retina ensures that visual cells respond mainly to luminance contrasts at the edges of stimuli and not to uniform illumination of the retina, Barlow, 1961); *orientation of edges* and *direction of movement*.

2. *Species-specific feature detectors.* Some classes of visual neuron are restricted to certain species and, in a teleological sense, might be concerned more with those particular elements of the visual environment that are especially relevant to the animal in question. The frog's bug detectors are a good example; so are the stereoscopic disparity detecting neurons in cat and monkey cortex; color sensitive cells in the goldfish (Wagner et al., 1960), the ground squirrel (Michael, 1968), and the monkey (Wiesel and Hubel, 1966); detectors of rotational movement in the fly (Mimura, 1970); these are all species-specific feature detectors, not found in every visual system.

The formation of feature-detecting neurons

This remarkable selectivity of visual neurons, whether for universal or for species-specific features, puts enormous demands on the anatomical construction of the animal's visual pathway. The properties of each cell depend on the precise nature of all the connections from the retinal rods and cones through to the neuron itself. It is difficult to believe that the staggering complexity of this circuitry could all be preprogrammed exactly by the genetic code.

Indeed it would be eminently reasonable (particularly for species-specific features) for the actual visual environment in which a developing visual system finds itself to play some part in sustaining, validating, or even specifying the connections that the visual system finally adopts.

In this chapter I shall present some evidence that early visual experience is crucially important for determining the feature-detecting properties of neurons in the cat's visual cortex. Early in a kitten's life, its vision is helping it to build a visual system appropriate to the world in which it lives.

The visual cortex of normal, adult cats

The primary visual cortex, in the occipital lobe, is just four synapses from the photoreceptors themselves. Hubel and Wiesel (1962) showed that, although the neurons in the cat's visual cortex are of several different kinds in their detailed properties, they are nearly all orientation selective and binocularly driven (Figure 1). Each cell responds

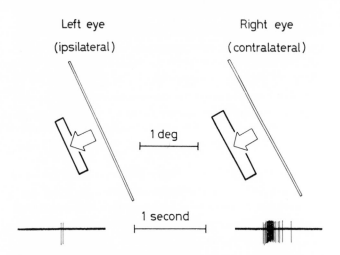

FIGURE 1 This binocular cortical neuron, recorded in the primary visual cortex of an adult cat, falls into ocular dominance group 2. The responses, in the records at the bottom photographed from an oscilloscope, show that a thin white bar moved across the receptive field (the thickly bordered rectangle) in the right eye is much more effective than the same stimulus shown to the left eye. (Reproduced, by permission, from Blakemore and Pettigrew, 1970.)

to a moving edge, or a light or dark bar, of a particular orientation, moving across the receptive field in either eye. The response is rapidly attenuated if the angle of the stimulus is altered (Figure 2). Different neurons prefer different orientations and, in the normal animal, every orientation is equally represented. Figure 3 is a polar diagram of the distribution of preferred orientations for a sample of neurons from the primary visual cortex of one

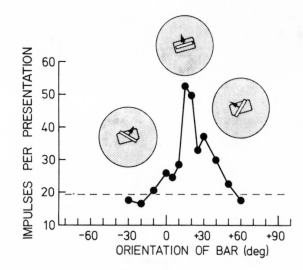

FIGURE 2 The orientational *tuning curve* for a *complex* cortical cell. The stimulus was a bright bar, generated on a display oscilloscope, as shown in the inset diagrams where the large rectangle is the receptive field. Each point is the mean number of impulses produced during six successive sweeps at that orientation. The dashed line is the mean spontaneous discharge in the same period of time, in the absence of any stimulus.

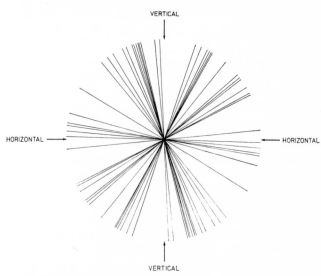

FIGURE 3 In this polar diagram, each line is the best orientation for one cortical neuron. This is a sample of 34 neurons from a normal adult cat.

cat. Each line is the best orientation for one cell; therefore, the cat has an armory of orientation detectors enabling it to deal with and analyze the shape of any object that it sees.

Although nearly all these cells are binocular, and they are almost certainly providing a mechanism for the recognition of stereoscopic distance (Barlow et al., 1967; Blakemore, 1970; Bishop, 1970), they are not all equally influenced by the two eyes. Hubel and Wiesel (1962) designed a simple qualitative scheme for categorizing the cells according to their ocular dominance (Figure 4),

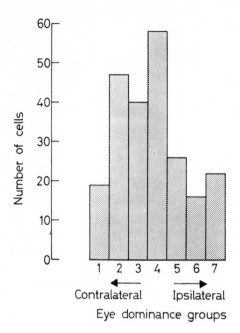

FIGURE 4 This histogram shows the distribution of ocular dominance among 228 cells from normal adult cats. The dominance groups describe the relative influence of the two eyes with group 4 cells being equally excited by the two eyes, group 1 cells driven only by the contralateral eye and group 7 cells only by the ipsilateral eye. (Reproduced, with permission, from Blakemore and Pettigrew, 1970.)

classifying them into seven dominance groups ranging from 1 (monocular cells only driven by the contralateral eye) through 4 (equally driven by both eyes) to 7 (monocular cells only driven by the ipsilateral eye).

The visual cortex of very young kittens

One obvious way of answering the whole question of the relative contributions of genetic and environmental factors would be to record from neurons in the visual cortex of very young kittens that have never had any visual experience. Both Hubel and Wiesel (1963) and Barlow and Pettigrew (1971) have studied young kittens and they agree about several things:

1. The neurons are inherently binocular with a normal ocular dominance distribution.

2. It is generally difficult to influence young cortical cells with visual stimuli; they respond very weakly and there is often rapid habituation during successive presentations of any stimulus.

3. A large number of cells certainly have *no* preference for any particular orientation and will respond equally for moving spots or edges of any angle.

There is strong disagreement about whether *any* cells are orientation detectors, like neurons in the adult. Hubel and Wiesel (1963) say there are many such cells; Barlow and Pettigrew (1971) say that there are none in the visually inexperienced kitten, although some are direction selective in the sense that they will respond to any target moving through the receptive field in a particular direction.

Therefore, some properties of cortical cells, such as their binocularity and their responses to movement, are certainly built in. Others seem to develop, or at least become sharpened up, during the first few weeks of vision. Now we must ask whether this process is passive maturation or whether it is a forceful influence of the environment.

Binocular deprivation

If both eyelids of a kitten are sutured shut at about 10 days of age (the time of natural eye opening) and its visual cortex is studied after several weeks of binocular deprivation, many of the neurons are still very infantile in their properties (Figure 5), many are not orientation selective, and a large number are completely visually unresponsive

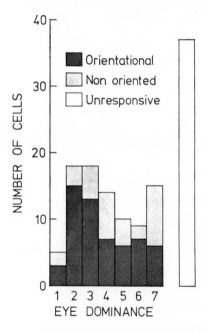

FIGURE 5 This ocular dominance histogram summarizes Wiesel and Hubel's experiments on binocular deprivation. There are 126 cells from 4 kittens deprived of vision from about 8 days until $2\frac{1}{2}$ to $4\frac{1}{2}$ months. Apparently normal orientation selective cells, cells with no orientational preference, and visually unresponsive neurons are shown separately. (From Blakemore, 1973.)

(Wiesel and Hubel, 1965). In fact, Barlow and Pettigrew (1971) maintain that a binocularly deprived cortex again has no orientation-selective cells at all. This certainly suggests that visual experience is essential for the establishment of the normal feature-detecting properties of neurons in the visual cortex and that they do not merely mature. On the other hand, the binocularity generally persists without any binocular visual experience.

Monocular deprivation

How different the result is if only one eyelid is closed during development. After such a period of monocular deprivation, the cortical cells that respond to visual stimuli can usually be influenced only through the experienced eye (Wiesel and Hubel, 1965). Apart from this monocular dominance, the cells are adult in their pattern-detecting properties.

These dramatic effects of monocular deprivation can occur only during a distinct *sensitive* or *critical period* (Figure 6). Covering one eye before the beginning of the

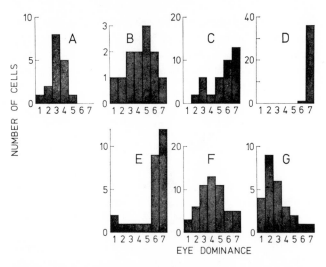

FIGURE 6   These histograms, redrawn from Hubel and Wiesel (1963, 1970b), illustrate the duration of the sensitive period for the results of monocular deprivation. (A) Results for two normal, very young, visually inexperienced kittens. In B to G the recordings were taken from the left hemisphere after the following periods of monocular deprivation in the right (contralateral) eye: (B) 9 to 19 days, (C) 10 to 31 days, (D) 23 to 29 days, (E) 2 to 3 months, (F) 4 to 7 months, (G) A previously normal adult monocularly deprived for 3 months. (From Blakemore, 1973.)

third week (Figure 6B) or after the fourth month (Figures 6F and 6G) has no influence on the dominance distribution; but as little as a few days of monocular deprivation during the fourth week (Figure 6D) leads to total dominance by the other eye (Hubel and Wiesel, 1970b).

During this remarkably short period, there must be intense competition for synaptic sites on cortical cells between the thalamocortical fibers from the two eyes, and it seems that simultaneous activity (or inactivity) in the two inputs is the requirement for the maintenance of binocular connections.

Environmental modification of orientation selectivity

If the degree of binocularity of cortical neurons can be influenced by visual experience, then possibly orientation selectivity itself can be modified by the visual environment. Hirsch and Spinelli (1971) combined the strategy of monocular deprivation with a procedure that dramatically limited the type of pattern that the cortex could experience. They reared kittens wearing an apparatus that allowed one eye to see three vertical lines, the other three horizontal ones. Thus the two eyes never saw similar orientations, and one might expect the binocularity of the cortex to suffer as a consequence. Indeed it did. All the cells with oriented receptive fields were monocular and all but one had a preferred orientation that closely matched the visual experience of the eye to which they were connected. There were no neurons, binocular or monocular, with diagonally-oriented receptive fields. This latter observation, and this alone, is incompatible with the simple notion that orientation selectivity is genetically specified and that there is merely competition between the inputs from the two eyes. If this were the case, all the diagonal detectors in Hirsch and Spinelli's cats should have been binocularly deprived, and therefore they should have survived. Because they did not, we must suspect that orientation selectivity itself can be *changed* by visual experience.

Blakemore and Cooper (1970) tested this idea with a much less sophisticated, but somewhat more naturalistic, apparatus. We reared two kittens in the dark except for a few hours each day when they were put into special chambers that essentially restricted their normal, binocular visual experience to edges of one orientation, vertical for one kitten, horizontal for the other (Figure 7). They stood on a glass plate suspended in a tall cylinder that was painted with black and white stripes and illuminated from above. A ruff around their necks prevented them from seeing their own bodies, so wherever they looked they simply saw stripes of one orientation.

The first two kittens had almost 300 hours of experience in this apparatus from 2 weeks to $5\frac{1}{2}$ months of age. After another 2 months, during which they were occasionally taken from the dark into a normal room to study their visual behavior, we recorded from the visual cortex of

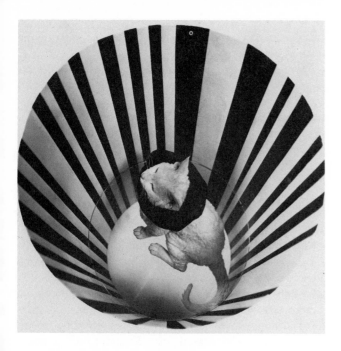

FIGURE 7   The apparatus for exposure to vertical edges. In this photograph the cat is almost full-grown.

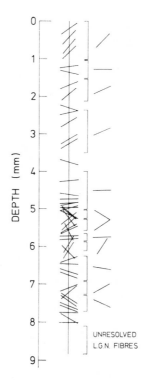

FIGURE 8   A reconstruction of the preferred orientations of neurons encountered during a long penetration through the visual cortex of a kitten reared in horizontal edges from 2 weeks to 5½ months. The columnar aggregates of cells with similar orientational preferences are shown by the bracketed regions on the right.

each animal. Despite their very strange early visual diet, we found virtually no visually unresponsive neurons or nonoriented cells and no regions of silent cortex. The neurons were quite normal and adult in their properties. Only one thing was really unusual: We could find no neurons that had a preferred orientation within 20 deg of the angle orthogonal to the stripes that the kitten had been reared in. Nearly all the cells responded best to orientations within 45 deg of that which the kitten had seen early in life.

Figure 8 is a reconstruction of a long penetration through the primary visual cortex of the first cat reared in horizontal stripes. The position of each neuron recorded in the penetration is shown by a line at the best orientation for that cell. Just as in the normal adult's cortex, neighboring neurons tended to prefer very similar orientations. These *columns* of cells are shown in Figure 8 as bracketed regions with the average preferred orientation for each column on the right.

There is, then, little doubt that early visual experience (albeit rather odd) can modify the orientation selectivity as well as the binocularity of cortical cells. By analogy with Wiesel and Hubel's hypothesis of competition between the inputs from the two eyes, one could imagine the newborn, naked cortical neuron besieged by groups of afferent fibers, each group representing a different orientation of edge on the retina. The set of input fibers most often used might win the battle for synaptic space.

The sensitive period for environmental modification

I have recently completed a series of similar experiments in which kittens were exposed to stripes for a limited period of time at different ages, in an attempt to define whether there is a crucial sensitive period for environmental modification of orientation selectivity, as there is for the effects of monocular deprivation. The results, illustrated in Figure 9, showed that there is such a sensitive period and that it coincides exactly with that for the modification of binocularity.

All but three of the kittens who produced the results of Figure 9 were kept in the dark until a particular age and then were exposed in a striped environment for 2 to 4 hours each day for a period of time from a few days to a few weeks. After the period of visual experience, they were kept continuously in the dark until I recorded from their cortical neurons, some days or weeks later. The abscissa of Figure 9 is the animal's age and each polar diagram is positioned at the kitten's age in the middle of the period of exposure. The upper half of Figure 9 shows kittens exposed to vertical stripes, the lower half those

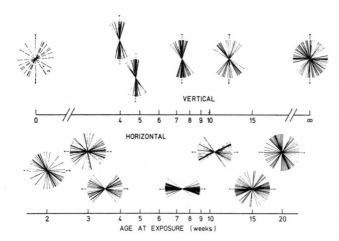

FIGURE 9 The critical period for environmental modification of the visual cortex. These kittens, with the exceptions described in the text, were kept in the dark and exposed to vertical (upper half) or horizontal (lower half) for a few hours each day, at various ages. On the upper abscissa the results that appear above zero age refer to a binocularly deprived kitten where the orientational preferences (dashed lines) were very vague, and those at ∞ on the abscissa are for a normal adult animal kept in vertical stripes over a 4 month period. The logarithmic abscissa carries no theoretical implications: It is merely for graphical convenience.

exposed to horizontal. The three exceptions to this basic paradigm are as follows:

1. The animal whose diagram lies above zero age on the upper abscissa had no visual experience. Its eyelids were sutured before natural eye opening and only re-opened just before the recording (Blakemore and Mitchell, 1972). This animal had many visually unresponsive and completely nonoriented neurons and even the cells illustrated in Figure 9 had only the merest bias toward the orientations shown. (That is why the lines are drawn interrupted rather than solid.) They all responded to some extent to every orientation of edge and almost as well for a moving spot. This kind of behavior is totally unlike that of adult neurons or indeed all the other cells shown in these polar diagrams. Therefore, on the basis of this very preliminary study, we must agree more with Barlow and Pettigrew (1971) than with Wiesel and Hubel (1965).

2. The kitten whose diagram appears at 15 weeks on the lower abscissa was kept in a normal lighted room until it was 6 weeks old, after which it was treated like all the others. This was done to preclude the possibility of simple degeneration due to disuse in the visual pathway during the long waiting period in the dark.

3. The results shown at ∞ on the upper abscissa refer to a normal adult cat that was kept in the dark for 4

months, during which it spent about 135 hours in the vertically striped environment.

From Figure 9 it is clear that the sensitivity to environmental modification increases suddenly at about 3 weeks of age, remains particularly high from 4 to 7 weeks, and then declines gradually, until after about 14 weeks of age no amount of experience of one orientation will influence the visual cortex.

However, kittens kept in the dark and exposed to stripes only before or after this critical period have many real orientation-selective neurons (quite unlike the binocularly deprived animal), even though there is no over representation of the experienced orientation. Two possible explanations spring to mind. Either there is another sensitive period, starting earlier and finishing later, during which *any* visual input will strengthen any innate predispositions in the neurons without modifying their preferences; or the few seconds of dim light that these kittens experienced each day in the dark room, during feeding and cleaning, was enough to set up many normal cortical cells, for all orientations.

The minimum necessary exposure

Even in the experiments described in Figure 9 the kittens were exposed for rather long periods of time, usually 30 to 50 hours, so one could argue that such a prolonged and unusual visual experience is so unlike a kitten's normal early vision that perhaps environmental modification is simply an artifact of a bizarre experimental manipulation. Blakemore and Mitchell (1973) very recently set out to define the minimum length of time in a striped environment that is necessary to influence the organization of the visual cortex.

We knew that the fourth week is a period of extraordinary sensitivity, so we kept six kittens in the usual manner and exposed them to vertical for various lengths of time (1, 3, 6, 18, 27, and 33 hours) on or around the 28th day and performed the recording at 6 weeks of age. The results, shown in Figure 10, surprised us and taught us that we had planned our experiment rather badly! The results for the binocularly deprived animal are reproduced (Figure 10A) for comparison, and it is patently clear that even 1 hour of vision totally changes the properties of the visual cortex. Not only were almost all the cells adult in their properties but the orientational preferences were mainly for angles close to vertical (Figure 10B). The few cells biased toward other orientations were generally more infantile in their properties, and we found them, together with a few nonoriented and visually unresponsive neurons, in small regions between the totally normal columns of cells that responded best to vertical.

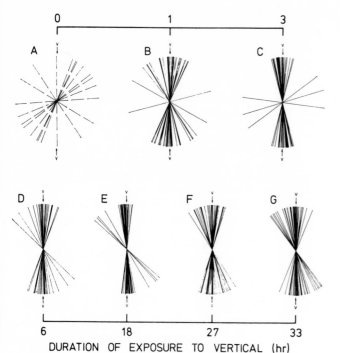

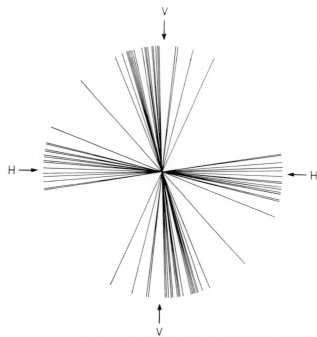

FIGURE 10 Orientational preferences for the cortical cells of six kittens (B to G) exposed to vertical for 1, 3, 6, 18, 27, and 33 hours, on or around the 28th day of age. The diagram with dashed lines (A) shows the vague orientational preferences of cells from a binocularly deprived kitten. (Reproduced, by permission, from Blakemore and Mitchell, 1973.)

FIGURE 11 The orientational preferences for 37 cells from a kitten exposed alternatively for 2 hours to horizontal, 2 hours to vertical, until it had experienced more than 50 hours of each.

There was a further slight refinement in the distribution of preferred orientations with longer exposure (Figures 10C to G), but the bulk of the process needs only 1 hour of experience.

An alternating visual environment

If 1 hour of vision is enough to modify cortical neurons, then what would be the effect of alternating exposure to the two orientations? Blakemore and Mitchell (in preparation) have allowed kittens to see horizontal and vertical stripes alternately, for various cycle lengths. Figure 11 shows what happened to the cortical neurons of a kitten reared for 2 hours in horizontal, 2 hours in vertical, 2 hours in horizontal, and so on, until it had accumulated more than 50 hours in each. It had two distinct populations of neurons, with their orientational preferences clustered around the two axes.

In general the columnar structure in this kitten, and others with a similar history, was as might be expected—columns of cells preferring vertical alternated with columns of neurons preferring horizontal orientation. However, there were also large regions of mixed orienta-

tion, with horizontal and vertical detecting neurons all jumbled up. In these strange columns we found some very peculiar cells: Some that were inhibited by one orientation and excited by the perpendicular, others that could not be excited and were only inhibited by one orientation, and still others that were excited by both axes (but not by diagonal edges) and, hence, responded best to a cross shape moving through the receptive field. These dual-axis cells are reminiscent of, but not identical to, Hubel and Wiesel's (1965) "higher-order hypercomplex cells" found only in area 19 of the cortex, not in area 17. Therefore, here is an indication that it is possible to synthesize feature-detecting neurons that are not normally found.

If, in such an alternating experiment, the *first* period of exposure comes in the fourth week and it lasts for 10 hours or more, it is difficult to reverse the arrangement by exposure to the opposite orientation, even for rather a long period. In such an animal, most cortical cells prefer the first orientation they experienced, and rather few are captured by the opposite.

Conclusions

Many questions about the genesis of the visual cortex remain unanswered. Is there, for instance, any contribution from the inbuilt predispositions of cortical cells?

Binocularity is innate, but it can certainly be modified. The position of the receptive field on the retina is also prewired, but even that is capable of being changed on the basis of visual experience (Shlaer, 1971).

Environmental modification becomes a simple phenomenon in the terribly reduced conditions of our experiments, but it is difficult to understand how it might operate in a normal kitten whose eye movements would expose each cortical cell to all orientations in quick succession. Perhaps it is merely the *probability* of experience that determines the final preference of a cell. Perhaps each neuron selects as its preferred stimulus the feature that it has seen most often. In that case environmental modification might have real adaptive value, because it would ensure that the animal builds for itself a visual system optimally matched to its particular visual world.

Humans have rather higher resolution acuity for vertical and horizontal patterns than for diagonal (Campbell, Kulikowski, and Levinson, 1966); perhaps this is due to the predominance of these orientations in the rectilinear environment of Western cities. More relevant, humans who grow up with astigmatism so severe that it greatly weakens the contrast of patterns of one orientation are left with "meridional amblyopia"—a reduced acuity for the orientation that was originally out of focus (Mitchell, Freeman, Millodot, and Haegerstrom, 1973). This meridional amblyopia, like normal reduced acuity for diagonals, cannot be rectified by perfect spectacle correction of the eye's optics.

Finally, it now seems valid to speculate that the actual physical changes that take place in the cortex during environmental modification are analogous to the fundamental process underlying learning and memory. We have no idea what is the physical correlate of, say, a visual memory of a complex object, but because total environmental modification of the visual cortex can occur after an hour or less of vision, it is worth considering the idea that memory itself depends on similar anatomical rearrangements to synthesize gnostic neurons in the brain.

ACKNOWLEDGMENTS G. F. Cooper and D. E. Mitchell collaborated in some of the experiments on the development of visual cortex. This work was generously supported by research grants (Nos. G970/807/B and G972/463/B) from the Medical Research Council, London. It would all have been impossible without the excellent technical assistance of R. D. Loewenbein and J. S. Dormer.

REFERENCES

BARLOW, H. B., 1961. Possible principles underlying the transformations of sensory messages. In *Sensory Communication*, W. A. Rosenblith, ed. Cambridge, Mass.: MIT Press, pp. 217–234.

BARLOW, H. B., and R. M. HILL, 1963. Selective sensitivity to direction of movement in ganglion cells of the rabbit retina. *Science* 139:412–414.

BARLOW, H. B., and J. D. PETTIGREW, 1971. Lack of specificity of neurones in the visual cortex of young kittens. *J. Physiol.* (*London*) 218:98–100P.

BARLOW, H. B., C. BLAKEMORE, and J. D. PETTIGREW, 1967. The neural mechanism of binocular depth discrimination. *J. Physiol.* (*London*) 193:327–342.

BISHOP, P. O., 1970. Beginning of form perception and binocular depth discrimination in cortex. In *The Neurosciences: Second Study Program*, F. O. Schmitt, ed. New York: Rockefeller University Press, pp. 471–485.

BLAKEMORE, C., 1970. The representation of three-dimensional visual space in the cat's striate cortex. *J. Physiol.* (*London*) 209:155–178.

BLAKEMORE, C., 1973. Environmental constraints on development in the visual system. In *Constraints on Learning: Limitations and Predispositions*, R. A. Hinde and J. S. Hinde, eds. London: Academic (in press).

BLAKEMORE, C., and G. COOPER, 1970. Development of the brain depends on the visual environment. *Nature* 228:477–478.

BLAKEMORE, C., and D. E. MITCHELL, 1973. Environmental modification of the visual cortex and the neural basis of learning and memory. *Nature* (in press).

BLAKEMORE, C., and J. D. PETTIGREW, 1970. Eye dominance in the visual cortex. *Nature* 225:426–429.

CAMPBELL, F. W., J. J. KULIKOWSKI, and J. LEVINSON, 1966. The effect of orientation on the visual resolution of gratings. *J. Physiol.* (*London*) 187:427–436.

HIRSCH, H. V. B., and D. N. SPINELLI, 1971. Modification of the distribution of receptive field orientation in cats by selective visual exposure during development. *Exp. Brain Res.* 12:509–527.

HUBEL, D. H., and T. N. WIESEL, 1962. Receptive fields, binocular interaction and functional architecture in the cat's visual cortex. *J. Physiol.* (*London*) 160:106–154.

HUBEL, D. H., and T. N. WIESEL, 1963. Receptive fields of cells in striate cortex of very young, visually inexperienced kittens. *J. Neurophysiol.* 26:994–1002.

HUBEL, D. H., and T. N. WIESEL, 1965. Receptive fields and functional architecture in two non-striate visual areas (18 and 19) of the cat. *J. Neurophysiol.* 28:229–289.

HUBEL, D. H., and T. N. WIESEL, 1970a. Cells sensitive to binocular depth in area 18 of the macaque monkey cortex. *Nature* 225:41–42.

HUBEL, D. H., and T. N. WIESEL, 1970b. The period of susceptibility to the physiological effects of unilateral eye closure in kittens. *J. Physiol.* (*London*) 206:419–436.

LETTVIN, J. Y., H. R. MATURANA, W. S. McCULLOCH, and W. H. PITTS, 1959. What the frog's eye tells the frog's brain. *Proc. Inst. Radio Engr.* 47:1940–1951.

LEVICK, W. R., 1967. Receptive fields and trigger features of ganglion cells in the visual streak of the rabbit's retina. *J. Physiol.* (*London*) 188:285–307.

MICHAEL, C. R., 1968. Receptive fields of single optic nerve fibers in a mammal with an all-cone retina. III: Opponent color units. *J. Neurophysiol.* 31:268–282.

MIMURA, K., 1970. Integration and analysis of movement information by the visual system of flies. *Nature* 226:964–966.

MITCHELL, D. E., R. D. FREEMAN, M. MILLODOT, and G. HAEGERSTROM, 1973. Meridional amblyopia: evidence for modification of the human visual system by early visual experience. *Vision Res.* (In press.)

MÜLLER, J., 1842. *Elements of Physiology*, Book V, Vol. II, translated by W. Baly. London: Taylor and Walton, pp. 1059–1087. (Reproduced in *Visual Perception: the Nineteenth Century*, W. Dember, ed. 1964. New York: John Wiley & Sons, pp. 35–69.)

SHLAER, R., 1971. Shift in binocular disparity causes compensatory change in the cortical structure of kittens. *Science* 173: 638–641.

WAGNER, H. G., E. F. MacNICHOL, and M. L. WOLBARSHT, 1960. The response properties of single ganglion cells in the goldfish retina. *J. Gen. Physiol.* 43 (Suppl. 2):45–62.

WIESEL, T. N., and D. H. HUBEL, 1965. Comparison of the effects of unilateral and bilateral eye closure on cortical unit responses in kittens. *J. Neurophysiol.* 28:1029–1040.

WIESEL, T. N., and D. H. HUBEL, 1966. Spatial and chromatic interactions in the lateral geniculate body of the rhesus monkey. *J. Neurophysiol.* 29:1115–1156.

11 Processing of Spatial and Temporal Information in the Visual System

MICHAEL J. WRIGHT and HISAKO IKEDA

ABSTRACT *On* center and *off* center receptive fields of cat retinal ganglion cells can be divided into two categories: *sustained* or *X-cells* and *transient* or *Y-cells*. The receptive field organization of the two categories of cells was investigated by several independent methods and found to differ. These results suggested that *X*- and *Y*-cells might begin the separate processing of spatial and temporal features of visual stimuli. Evidence is presented that the information from *X*- and *Y*-cells is transmitted over separate central pathways, and that the thresholds for detection of spatial and temporal contrast are set by different populations of neurons.

Introduction

SEVERAL SOURCES of evidence suggest that the visual pathways contain neurons that are specifically tuned to different stimuli of submodalities, for example, orientation, size, and retinal disparity.

On the other hand, examination of the receptive field organization of retinal ganglion cells in the cat reveals two basic types, *sustained* and *transient* cells. This paper considers evidence that these two classes of retinal ganglion cells are the origin for the *separate* processing of spatial and temporal features of visual stimuli, respectively, and that the submodalities of vision may be grouped around this spatial/temporal dichotomy.

Retinal ganglion cell receptive fields in the cat

The classical description of the receptive field of the cat's retinal ganglion cell was given by Kuffler (1953). Within each receptive field, he described a central area with a low threshold to a small, flashing spot of light. The discharge pattern of this center region is opposite to that found in the surround or periphery. The center may give predominantly *off*, the surround *on* discharges, or vice

versa. The familiar concentric arrangement of receptive field regions revealed by plotting the field with a small spot of light is shown in Figure 1(a).

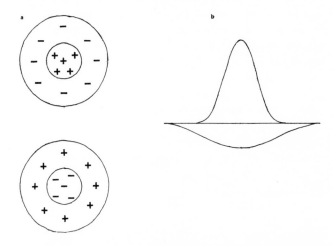

FIGURE 1   (a) Receptive field of an on-center (top) and an off-center (bottom) retinal ganglion cell as revealed by plotting with a small spot of light. The concentric, center-surround organization described by Kuffler (1953) is shown. (b) Model of retinal ganglion cell receptive field proposed by Rodieck (1965). The *X*-axis shows distance along a diameter of the receptive field, and the *Y*-axis shows sensitivity. Center and surround mechanisms have concentric, overlapping, Gaussian sensitivity distributions, the peak sensitivity of the surround being smaller than that of the center and its variance greater. The center and surround mechanisms sum their inputs separately and have opposite, antagonistic effects on the ganglion cell discharge. The model applies both to on-center and to off-center cells.

A receptive field plot of this kind is the result of a particular experimental procedure: It is obtained with a spot of particular diameter and intensity, rather than being a constant property of the cell. The receptive field plot alone does not permit a full prediction of the response of the cell to other visual stimuli. Indications of this fact were evident in the original experiments of Kuffler (1953), who

MICHAEL J. WRIGHT and HISAKO IKEDA   Research Department of Ophthalmology, Royal College of Surgeons of England, London, England

found that the spatial extent of the receptive field increased when the intensity of the plotting spot was increased. Similarly, Ikeda and Wright (1972a) showed that the field expands if the area of the spot is increased while its intensity is kept constant. The obvious interpretation of these findings is that spots of greater intensity or area stimulate additional regions of lower sensitivity, so that a complete description of the receptive field must include the *spatial distribution of sensitivity* of the center and surround.

A model of this type, developed from Kuffler's findings, has been proposed by Rodieck (1965) (see Figure 1(b)). It assumes that the distributions of the center and surround sensitivities are Gaussian, concentric, and overlapping, with the surround distribution having a smaller peak and larger variance. Signals from photoreceptors in the center region and signals from photoreceptors in the surround region are summed separately, and the resulting signals have opposite, antagonistic effects on the ganglion cell response. In other words, there is linear spatial summation in both center and surround, and a subtractive interaction. This model applies both to on-center and to off-center fields.

In accord with this model, a luminance increment within the field will produce a response, either excitatory or inhibitory: But if the luminance changes in symmetrical halves of the field are equal and opposite, the signals reaching the cell from each half of the center and surround mechanism will be equal and opposite, giving no net response. This test of Rodieck's model was carried out by Enroth-Cugell and Robson (1966). One class of retinal ganglion cells (*X*-cells) behaved according to the model, but for another group (*Y*-cells) there was no null position of the stimulus border within the receptive field. This was not due to radial asymmetry of *Y*-cell fields, because they, too, have the concentric organization described by Kuffler (1953) but resulted from some form of nonlinearity of spatial summation. (A model of the *Y*-cell receptive field has recently been proposed by Ikeda and Wright, 1972b).

The *X/Y* classification, therefore, reflects a fundamental difference in receptive field organization; it is not dependent on a particular method of plotting the field. Cleland, Dubin, and Levick (1971) showed that *X*- and *Y*-cells also differed in their response to a small steady spot of appropriate contrast to excite the receptive field center.

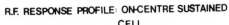

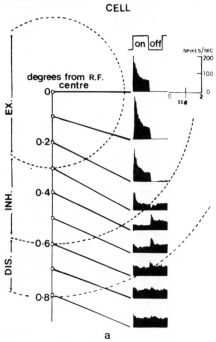
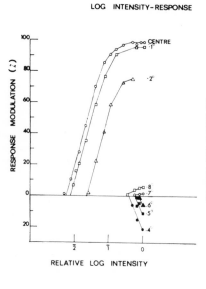
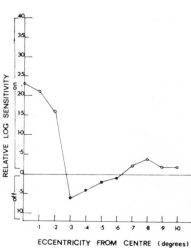

a   b   c

FIGURE 2   (a) Poststimulus histograms obtained from an on-center sustained cell at different distances from the receptive field center (0°–0.8°). The locations of the excitatory center and the inhibitory and outer excitatory surrounds are shown diagramatically. Spot size 25′, spot intensity 257 cd/m², background intensity 17.5 cd/m². (b) Response as a function of log intensity of the stimulus at different distances from the receptive field center. Unattenuated spot intensity, size, and background intensity as in Figure 2a. Note that the *off* response also shows a linear response to log intensity. (c) Sensitivity gradient of the cell derived from Figure 2b by reading off the intensity level required to produce a threshold response for each location. (From Ikeda and Wright, 1972c,d.)

The responses of Y-cells are phasic; there is a transient excitation when the spot is introduced which decays, in 5 sec or less, to a steady maintained level. In the X-cell response, however, there is a tonic component while the spot is present. On the basis of their response to a steady contrast, X- and Y-cells are also known by the descriptive names, *sustained* and *transient* cells (Cleland, Dubin, and Levick, 1971). In the following, we use the terms sustained and transient to refer to cells showing behavior characteristic of X- and Y-cells.

Receptive field organization of sustained and transient cells

In order to obtain a more complete characterization of ganglion cell behavior, we plotted the receptive field of each cell repeatedly, using spots of different diameters and a wide range of intensities extending to threshold. This method enabled us to determine both sensitivity gradients and spatial summation properties across the receptive fields of sustained and transient cells.

Figure 2 shows the results of a basic experiment of this type, for a single on-center sustained cell; Figure 2(a) shows the change in the poststimulus histogram as the spot position is moved from the excitatory center to the inhibitory surround. Beyond the inhibitory surround, we found in nearly all cells by averaging of the responses a small peak of excitation that constituted an outer excitatory (disinhibitory) surround (Ikeda and Wright, 1972c). Figure 2(b) shows the effect of varying the intensity of the spot. When we plotted the logarithm of the spot intensity against the percentage response modulation, we obtained a linear response at low intensities and a saturation at high intensities. The inhibitory surround and outer excitatory surround also have approximately a linear response to log spot intensity. Figure 2(c) shows the sensitivity gradient plotted from this data.

In Figure 3, the same experiment is carried out on an on-center transient cell. The poststimulus histograms obtained at different positions across the receptive field (with approximately the same stimulating conditions used in Figure 2) are shown in Figure 3(a). The histograms

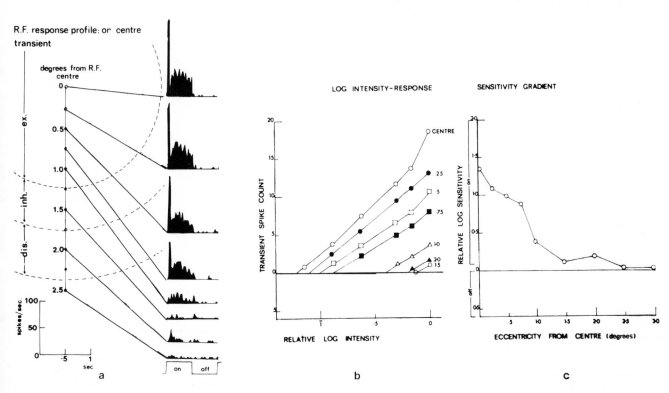

a

b

c

FIGURE 3 (a) Poststimulus histograms obtained from an on-center transient cell at different distances (0°–2.5°) from the receptive field center. The approximate locations of the excitatory center, inhibitory, and outer excitatory surrounds are shown diagramatically, but the divisions are in fact ill-defined. Spot size 28', spot intensity 230 cd/m², background intensity 10 cd/m². No distinctive response is obtained from the inhibitory surround with this stimulus. (b) Response of this cell as a function of log spot intensity at different distances from the

receptive field center. Unattenuated spot intensity, size, and background intensity as in Figure 3a. The transition from the inhibitory to the outer excitatory zone appears as a reverse order of response-intensity curves at 1.5° and 2.0°. (c) Sensitivity gradient of the cell derived from Figure 3b, by reading off the intensity level required to produce threshold response at each location. (From Ikeda and Wright, 1972c, and unpublished data.)

have a characteristically different shape, with a very brief initial excitation. There is only a very small off response from the surround, and this co-exists with a much larger center-type response. The on response increases again beyond the inhibitory surround in the outer excitatory region. In Figure 3(b), the response/log intensity function is shown for different receptive field locations, and Figure 3(c) shows the sensitivity gradient reconstructed from this data. Unlike sustained cells, transient cells rarely showed a clear division of the sensitivity gradient into excitatory, inhibitory, and outer excitatory zones, because the surround did not give an appreciable response, its threshold to spot stimulation being 1–2 log units higher than that of sustained cells. If a larger spot was used, a clear surround response appeared. This is shown in Figure 4.

In transient cells, however, if the stimulus spot were enlarged so as to elicit a surround response, the center response was increased also. It was rarely possible to elicit a pure surround response in transient cells, because the receptive field center expands with increased stimulus flux (Ikeda and Wright, 1972a), and transient, on-off responses are then obtained from points in the field periphery (Figure 4). In sustained cells, this did not occur. There was always a diminution of the response if the spot were enlarged beyond a certain size, due to center-surround antagonism, and a definite limit to the expansion of the receptive field center with increasing spot size (Ikeda and Wright, 1972a).

The results of this series of experiments may be summarized under four headings.

First, we confirmed the observation of Cleland, Dubin, and Levick (1971) that transient cells gave strongly phasic responses while sustained cells gave tonic responses with an initial phasic component to a small spot in the receptive field center. Furthermore, the phasic response of transient cells was maintained throughout the receptive field, whereas the tonic response of sustained cells tended to decrease with increasing eccentricity (Ikeda and Wright, 1972d).

Second, we found that the antagonism of center and surround was much stronger in sustained than in transient cells. In sustained cells the regions from which mixed on-off discharges could be obtained were limited to the boundaries between excitatory and inhibitory regions, whereas in transient cells, a transient center-type response often persisted throughout the entire surround.

Third, we have shown that sustained cells had an optimum spot size beyond which the cell response decreased, whereas there was no marked decrease in response for larger-than-optimum stimuli in transient cells. The expansion of the receptive field with increasing spot size in transient cells (Figure 4) was associated with the presence of a periphery effect (McIlwain, 1964), which

R.F. response profile; on-centre transient

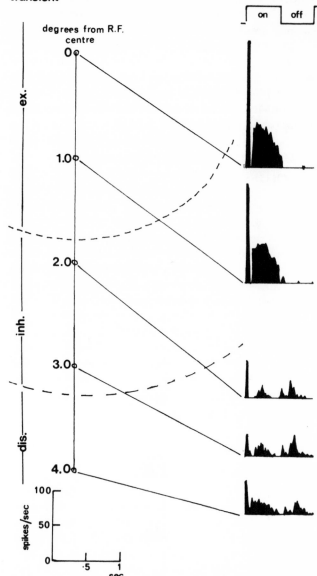

FIGURE 4 Poststimulus histograms obtained at different locations in the receptive field of an on-center transient cell. This is the same cell as shown in Figure 3, but the stimulus spot is larger (51′). Other stimulus conditions as in Figure 3. The excitatory, inhibitory, and outer excitatory zones all show an apparent increase in diameter with the larger spot, and a definite off response is obtained from the inhibitory surround, but there is still considerable overlap between receptive field zones, and mixed (on-off) responses are obtained from most of the receptive field periphery (Ikeda and Wright, unpublished observations.)

we have argued is an extension of receptive field properties into the far periphery. (Ikeda and Wright, 1972b).

Fourth, the spatial extent of the excitatory, inhibitory, and disinhibitory phases of the sensitivity gradient was greater in transient than in sustained cells. If the diameter of the sensitivity gradient were taken at $1/e$ of the sensitivity of the central point, the mean value was 0.7° for sustained cells at 3–8° from the area centralis, while it was 2.1° for transient cells from the same retinal region. The surrounds of transient cells were also larger than those of sustained cells by a factor of 3. A similar result was obtained by Cleland and Levick (1972).

Given these receptive field properties, we can make some generalizations about the types of visual information transmitted by sustained and transient cells. With their narrow, sharply peaked sensitivity gradients, sustained cells are able to resolve finer visual detail than transient cells. It is known that sustained cells preserve information about the phase of the finest resolvable grating patterns drifting across the receptive field whereas transient cells respond only to the onset and offset of movement of such gratings (Enroth-Cugell and Robson, 1966). The smaller surround diameter of sustained cells gives them sharper tuning to stimulus size. Although the response of transient cells is less critically dependent on the spatial distribution of illumination in the receptive field, the phasic nature of the response gives greater temporal definition than the tonic responses of sustained cells. Sustained cells would therefore seem to be concerned predominantly with the spatial aspects of visual stimuli, and transient cells with the temporal aspects.

Anatomical and physiological independence of sustained and transient pathways

The sustained/transient classification of visual neurons corresponds to classifications based on other physiological or anatomical criteria. The fastest-conducting fibers in the cat's optic nerve are the axons of Y-cells, and the axons of X-cells are slower conducting (Cleland, Dubin, and Levick, 1971; Fukada, 1971). In addition, there is a group of very slow-conducting fibers, W-cells (Hoffmann and Stone, 1972), which have suppressed-by-contrast (Stone and Fabian, 1966), or excited-by-contrast receptive fields.

The destinations of these fiber groups within the central nervous system are different. The lateral geniculate nucleus (LGN) receives X- and Y-cell afferents (Cleland, Dubin, and Levick, 1971) whereas the superior colliculus receives W- and Y-cell fibers (Hoffmann and Stone, 1972). Moreover, as Cleland, Dubin, and Levick (1971) showed, cells within the LGN may be classified as sustained or transient on the same criteria as retinal ganglion cells; transient LGN cells receive their excitatory input *only* from transient optic nerve axons, and sustained LGN cells only from sustained optic nerve axons (Hoffmann, Stone, and Sherman, 1972). There is thus little mixing of

sustained and transient information arriving at the visual cortex.

Hoffmann and Stone (1971) present preliminary evidence that sustained and transient optic radiation axons innervate different populations of cortical neurons. However the classificatory scheme for cortical receptive fields that they used (the simple, complex, and hypercomplex cells of Hubel and Wiesel, 1965) must be extended to include the *temporal* as well as the *spatial* organization of receptive fields if the fate of sustained and transient inputs to the cortex is to be understood. Noda, Freeman, Gies, and Creutzfeldt (1971), who recorded from visual cortex neurons in awake, unparalyzed cats, found a large group of neurons giving tonic responses to stationary gratings in a preferred orientation, and found a second group that responded only when the grating was moved at moderate speed in a preferred direction; it would certainly be consistent with the known properties of neurons in the visual pathway to suppose that the motion-sensitive units received inputs from transient LGN cells and that units responding to stationary stimuli received sustained inputs.

The lateral posterior nucleus (LP) of the cat thalamus contains two visual centers, one of which receives fibers from the superior colliculus, the other from the visual cortex (see Ann Graybiel, Part 3 of this volume). Neurons in both regions are characterized by phasic responses, and many respond to discontinuous rather than smooth movements: They appear to be higher-order, movement-sensitive neurons of various kinds (Wright, 1971). The responses of a discontinuous movement unit from the lateral (cortical) part of LP are shown in Figure 5. The response characteristics of these neurons and the pattern of their afferent connections suggest that these cells are driven by transient neurons in visual cortex or superior colliculus.

This anatomical and physiological evidence points to the conclusion that there are separate sustained and transient pathways within the visual projections. Apparently the sustained pathway is limited to the geniculo-striate system, but the transient pathway has both cortical and subcortical branches and may subserve a corresponding multiplicity of functions.

There are differences in the distribution of sustained and transient ganglion cells across the retina. According to Cleland and Levick (1972), 90% of the cells in the area centralis were sustained and 10% transient, but for the remainder of the retinal area within 30° of the cat's area centralis, 62% were sustained and 38% transient. Ikeda and Wright (1972a) found that the proportion of transient cells increased steadily toward the periphery. The differing functions of the fovea and retinal periphery might be served by the filtering properties of sustained and transient

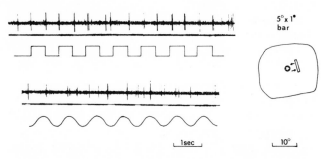

Square and sinusoidal movement

FIGURE 5 Response of a neuron in the lateral part of the lateral posterior nucleus (LP) of the cat to different modes of stimulus movement. In the upper trace, a 5° × 1° light rectangle is subjected to abrupt displacements of position within the receptive field (the rectangle is reflected off a mirror driven by a square wave of 1 Hz from a function generator). The neuron responds to each displacement of the rectangle with a short burst of spikes. In the lower trace, the rectangle is given a sinusoidal motion of the same frequency, and the cell no longer responds. Many units in LP showed this pattern of response, responding to discontinuous but not to smooth movements. (Wright, unpublished observations.)

cells. Transient cells are exquisitely sensitive to changes in the pattern of illumination over their receptive fields, such as may be produced by a moving object in the peripheral visual field. Attention-getting stimuli, which invariably involve such changes, initiate fixation reflexes resulting in the object of interest being centered on the fovea, where its spatial detail may be analyzed by the sustained pathway. Transient cells, particularly peripheral ones, are tolerant to defocusing of the stimulus by refractive errors (in a three-dimensional world, only objects lying along the visual axes are consistently kept in focus by accommodation), but central, sustained cells require a sharply focused image in order to respond (Ikeda and Wright, 1972a).

Role of sustained and transient cells in visual perception

In deciding the relevance of these arguments to general problems of visual perception, there are two questions to be answered. First, to what extent are findings in the cat characteristic of other species? Second, do the functional interpretations we have placed on the behavior of *X*- and *Y*-cells represent truly distinct modes of visual processing that can be identified in psychophysical experiments?

There is good evidence from comparative anatomy and physiology that the sustained/transient classification is applicable to the visual pathways of a wide range of vertebrates. Werblin and Dowling (1969) recorded sustained and transient retinal ganglion cells in *Necturus* and

identified amacrine cells as the element in the input network of ganglion cells responsible for the generation of transient responses. Dubin (1970) examined the inner plexiform layer of vertebrate retinas by electron microscopy and found greater number and complexity of amacrine synaptic connections in those species that have ganglion cells with refined temporal discrimination. Movement-sensitive ganglion cells may often be classified as transient on the basis of their response to a stationary spot, and a large majority of ganglion cells in the retina of the pigeon (L. Holden, unpublished results) and rabbit (H. Ikeda, unpublished results) are transient on the usual criteria; these species have a larger number of complex amacrine synapses than animals that rely on stereoscopic vision, such as the cat and monkey (Dubin, 1970).

Sustained and transient neurons also exist in primate visual systems. Gouras (1969) found that in the monkey retina, transient cells, as in the cat, have faster-conducting axons than sustained cells and are relatively more common in peripheral retina. In addition, transient cells mix signals from different cone mechanisms in both center and surround, but sustained cells receive excitatory signals from one cone mechanism in the center, and inhibitory signals from another cone mechanism in the periphery of the receptive field (Gouras, 1968).

The use of stimuli of spatially periodic patterns (gratings) with variable contrast and constant mean luminance, and the application of Fourier analysis to the results, have considerably advanced the psychophysics of form perception (Campbell, earlier in this part). The same methods may be extended to include temporal periodicities in stimuli, and some investigations of this type do provide evidence that spatial and temporal features of visual stimuli are to some extent separately encoded in the nervous system.

Kulikowski (1971) used a sinusoidal grating, of variable spatial frequency, that was alternated 180° in phase at temporal frequencies of 0.5–30 Hz, and viewed monocularly, with central fixation. At intermediate spatial and temporal frequencies, such a grating is in apparent movement appearing to drift in either direction at constant speed. However, if the spatial frequency were above 20 c/deg, Kulikowski's subjects reported that the grating appeared to be stationary. When the contrast of the grating was varied, it was found that the threshold for detecting the grating was lower than the threshold for detecting the apparent movement, at all spatial frequencies. As this experiment proves, it is possible to detect a grating without being aware of its movement, whereas as soon as a grating is above threshold contrast, the subject is aware of its orientation and spatial frequency.

A plausible explanation for this phenomenon is that even for patterns stimulating the central retina, the detection of purely spatial (orientation and spatial frequency) features and the detection of spatiotemporal (real and apparent movement) features of stimuli are accomplished by different mechanisms, which might be elements in the sustained and transient pathways, respectively. The low sensitivity of the transient pathway to patterns of high spatial frequency and low contrast would prevent its stimulation by such patterns, resulting in elimination of the sensation of movement, while the sustained pathway continued to detect the grating itself.

Experiments by Pantle and Sekuler (1969) support the conclusion that the detection of stationary patterns and of movement is accomplished by separate mechanisms. They found that prolonged viewing of a slowly moving grating of high contrast led to a reduction in contrast sensitivity for specific test targets. By varying the contrast of the adapting grating, they separated two components of the response. The first was specific to the orientation of the grating and was independent of its movement, and the second was specific to the direction of movement. The orientation- and direction-specific mechanisms revealed in these experiments showed different changes in contrast sensitivity with an adapting stimulus of equal contrast and duration.

There is evidence that many purely spatial features of visual stimuli are encoded by a *single* population of cells: Detectors that are tuned to spatial frequency are also orientation specific (Blakemore and Campbell, 1969) and even specific for retinal disparity (Blakemore and Hague, 1972). Blakemore (1973) suggests that each cortical cell encodes a variety of (spatial) submodalities and that a single cortical cell is thus *multichannel* in nature, so that the same population of cells would encode *all* the orientations, *all* the spatial frequencies, and *all* the disparities.

On the other hand, the psychophysical experiments reviewed here would suggest that *different* populations of cells are concerned with the detection of a pattern and the detection of its movement. It would appear that for central vision, there are at least two populations of cells in the brain, one encoding the spatial features of stimuli, the other encoding movement. The characteristics of this second population of cells, which presumably receives input from transient neurons, and the role of transient cells in peripheral vision are in need of further investigation.

ACKNOWLEDGMENTS   The work in this laboratory was supported by the Medical Research Council and the R.N.I.B. We thank Janet Nuza, Sheena Dyer and John Dench for excellent technical assistance. The experiments on the lateral posterior nucleus by M. J. Wright were done in the Psychological Laboratory, Cambridge, and supported by the Medical Research Council. Thanks are due to Dr. G. Horn for help at all stages of this work.

REFERENCES

BLAKEMORE, C., 1973. Central visual processing. In *Foundations of Psychobiology*, M. S. Gazzaniga and C. Blakemore, eds. London and New York: Academic Press.

BLAKEMORE, C., and F. W. CAMPBELL, 1969. On the existence in the human visual system of neurons selectively sensitive to the orientation and size of retinal images. *J. Physiol. (London)* 203:237–260.

BLAKEMORE, C., and B. HAGUE, 1972. Evidence for disparity-detecting neurons in the human visual system. *J. Physiol. (London)* 225:437–456.

CLELAND, B. G., M. W. DUBIN, and W. R. LEVICK, 1971. Sustained and transient neurons in the cat retina and lateral geniculate nucleus. *J. Physiol. (London)* 217:473–497.

CLELAND, B. G., and W. R. LEVICK, 1972. Physiology of cat retinal ganglion cells. *Invest. Ophthal.* 11:285–290.

DUBIN, M. W., 1970. The inner plexiform layer of the retina: a quantitative and comparative electron microscopic analysis. *J. Comp. Neurol.* 140:479–506.

ENROTH-CUGELL, C., and J. G. ROBSON, 1966. The contrast sensitivity of retinal ganglion cells of the cat. *J. Physiol. (London)* 187:517–552.

FUKADA, Y., 1971. Receptive field organization of cat optic nerve fibers with special reference to conduction velocity. *Vision Res.* 11:209–226.

GOURAS, P., 1968. Identification of cone mechanisms in monkey ganglion cells. *J. Physiol. (London)* 199:533–547.

GOURAS, P., 1969. Antidromic responses of orthodromically identified ganglion cells in monkey retina. *J. Physiol. (London)* 204:407–419.

HOFFMANN, K.-P., and J. STONE, 1971. Conduction velocity of afferents to cat visual cortex: a correlation with cortical receptive field properties. *Brain Res.* 32:460–466.

HOFFMAN, K.-P., J. STONE, and M. SHERMAN, 1972. Relay of receptive field properties in dorsal lateral geniculate nucleus of the cat. *J. Neurophysiol.* 35:518–531.

HUBEL, D. H., and T. N. WIESEL, 1962. Receptive fields, binocular interaction and functional architecture in the cat's visual cortex. *J. Physiol. (London)* 160:106–154.

HUBEL, D. H., and T. N. WIESEL, 1965. Receptive fields, binocular interaction and functional architecture in two non-striate visual areas (18 and 19) of the cat. *J. Neurophysiol.* 28:229–289.

IKEDA, H., and M. J. WRIGHT, 1972a. Differential effects of refractive errors and receptive field organization of central and peripheral ganglion cells. *Vision Res.* 12:1465–1476.

IKEDA, H., and M. J. WRIGHT, 1972b. Functional organization of the periphery effect in retinal ganglion cells. *Vision Res.* 12:1857–1879.

IKEDA, H., and M. J. WRIGHT, 1972c. The outer disinhibitory surround of the retinal ganglion cell receptive field. *J. Physiol. (London)* 226:511–544.

IKEDA, H., and M. J. WRIGHT, 1972d. Receptive field organization of "sustained" and "transient" retinal ganglion cells which subserve different functional roles. *J. Physiol. (London)* 227:769–800.

KUFFLER, S. W., 1953. Discharge patterns and functional organization of the mammalian retina. *J. Neurophysiol.* 16:37–68.

KULIKOWSKI, J. J., 1971. Effect of eye movements on the contrast sensitivity of spatio-temporal patterns. *Vision Res.* 11:261–273.

McILWAIN, J. T., 1964. Receptive fields of optic tract axons and lateral geniculate neurons: peripheral extent and barbiturate sensitivity. *J. Neurophysiol.* 27:1154–1173.

NODA, H., R. B. FREEMAN, JR., B. GIES, and O. D. CREUTZFELDT, 1971. Neuronal responses in the visual cortex of awake cats to stationary and moving targets. *Exp. Brain Res.* 12:389–405.

PANTLE, A., and R. SEKULER, 1969. Contrast response of human visual mechanisms sensitive to orientation and direction of motion. *Vision Res.* 9:397–406.

RODIECK, R. W., 1965. Quantitative analysis of cat retinal ganglion cell response to visual stimuli. *Vision Res.* 5:583–601.

STONE, J., and M. FABIAN, 1966. Specialized receptive fields of the cat's retina. *Science* 152:1277–1279.

STONE, J., and K.-P. HOFFMANN, 1972. Very slow-conducting ganglion cells in the cat's retina: a major, new functional type? *Brain Res.* 43:610–616.

WERBLIN, F. S., and J. E. DOWLING, 1969. Organization of the retina of the mudpuppy, *Necturus maculosus*. II. Intracellular recording. *J. Neurophysiol.* 32:339–355.

WRIGHT, M. J., 1971. Responsiveness to visual stimuli of single neurons in the pulvinar and lateral posterior nuclei of the cat's thalamus. *J. Physiol.* (*London*) 219:32–33P.

12 The Psychophysics of Visually Induced Perception of Self-Motion and Tilt

JOHANNES DICHGANS and TH. BRANDT

ABSTRACT Visual stimuli that move in a horizontal plane may lead to two different perceptual interpretations: The observer may perceive himself either as being stationary in space while the visual stimulus appears to move or he may experience an illusion of self-motion while the moving surround appears at rest. Furthermore, when an observer views a wide-angled display rotating around his line of sight, he feels his body tilted and sees a vertical straight edge tilted in the direction opposite to the moving stimulus. Psychophysical and neurophysiological observations suggest that the sensation of optokinetically induced self-motion and tilt are attributable to interactions of visual and vestibular inputs within the vestibular system.

Introduction

A SUBJECT exposed to a large horizontally moving pattern may experience an apparent self-motion in the direction opposite to that of the moving visual stimulus (Mach, 1885; Helmholtz, 1896; Fischer and Kornmüller, 1930; Gurnee, 1931). At the same time, the moving pattern may seem to be stationary in space. This compelling illusion will invariably occur if the entire visual surroundings are moving and if enough time is allowed for stimulation. With stimulation in a horizontal plane, the perceived self-motion, which in the following will be called circular vection (CV), cannot be distinguished subjectively from true passive body motion (Brandt et al., 1971). This holds even with respect to *Coriolis effects* which, during real body rotation, are caused by bending the head toward the shoulder. Vestibular Coriolis effects are generally assumed to be mainly due to the effects of cross-coupling of angular acceleration applied to different semi-circular canals (Groen, 1961). Therefore, it is quite puzzling that during the visually induced illusion of self-rotation *pseudo-Coriolis effects* arise from similar head movements, which eventually lead to motion sickness. Their symptoms (apparent tilt, dizziness, drowsiness, and nausea) have been shown to be qualitatively the same as in Coriolis effects (Dichgans and

JOHANNES DICHGANS and TH. BRANDT   Department of Neurology, University of Freiburg, West Germany; Department of Psychology, Massachusetts Institute of Technology, Cambridge, Massachusetts.

Brandt, 1972).

A second phenomenon also underscores in our opinion the importance of visual motion information for orientation with respect to gravity: If exposed to a visual pattern that rotates in a vertical plane around the observer's line of sight, the subject will not only experience body motion but also tilt of both the visual and postural vertical (Dichgans et al., 1972). Similar observations have been made by Wood (1895) and Helmholtz (1896).

In this paper, both phenomena will be described in more detail. In each case, the role of stimulus time, stimulus velocity, and stimulus area and its location within the visual field will be examined. Special emphasis will be given to clarification of the stimulus features that determine whether or not a visual stimulus is perceived as moving in the outer world (egocentric motion perception) and that determine the perceived orientation of the body in space (exocentric motion perception).

Some of the results described in this paper led us to the assumption of visual-vestibular interaction within the vestibular system. Among these are the phenomenal equality of self-motion as perceived either by exclusive visual or by vestibular stimulation, the existence of pseudo-Coriolis effects, and the direction-specific modulation of vestibular thresholds (Young et al., 1972) for the perception of body acceleration during CV. The hypothesis will be discussed in reference to supporting evidence from a few neurophysiological experiments.

We feel justified in putting so much emphasis on these *illusions*, as they must be called under our experimental conditions, because the underlying physiological mechanisms participate in spatial orientation under real-life conditions. This will be shown in the last paragraph of the chapter.

Visually induced perception of self-motion

The *experimental apparatus* consisted of a rotating chair located in the center of a closed cylindrical drum 1.5 m in diameter whose inner walls were painted with alternating vertical black-and-white stripes subtending 7° of visual angle. Both the chair and the drum could be rotated separately or simultaneously in either the same or opposite directions and at the same or different speeds. Optokinetic stimulation by the moving drum could be restricted to any desirable spatial extent and could be presented at any location within the visual field. This was achieved by using black masks that were mounted immediately adjacent to the inner wall of the drum. The masks were fixed on poles connected to the back of the chair. To stabilize the direction of the visual axis, subjects were asked to focus on a 1° luminous spot mounted on the chair and presented in a position straight ahead of the subject. Eye movements were recorded by electronystagmography. In the different experiments described, a total of 68 students, who were previously unfamiliar with the investigated phenomena, took part in the study.

The *prolonged time course* of CV after onset and termination of the visual stimulus was studied with constant speeds of drum-rotation ranging between 10° and 180°/sec. Subjects initially sitting in the dark were suddenly exposed to the moving pattern (in the light) that stimulated the entire visual field. Invariably, the initial experience was that of surround motion; however, within an average of 3 to 4 sec, an apparent body acceleration opposite to the direction of drum-rotation began, during which the

surroundings seemed to move progressively more slowly. Within an average of 8 to 12 sec after stimulus onset, an exclusive self-rotation (CV) was perceived, and the surroundings seemed to be stationary. After switching off the illumination inside the drum, CV never stopped immediately but continued in the same direction, outlasting the visual stimulus by an average of 8 to 11 sec. The time course of CV shows considerable interindividual variability but is relatively constant for each subject over trials. In our experiments, latencies are barely influenced by stimulus velocities. This observation, and the fact that even with drum accelerations up to 15°/sec² subjects still experienced self-rotation, show that one cannot infer from the lack of actual vestibular stimulation that only the visual surround is moving.

The *velocity range* in which the sensation of exclusive self-motion can be elicited by a moving visual stimulus has its upper limit at approximately 90°/sec (Figure 1). Within this range, the perceived velocity of CV is linearly related to stimulus speed, and the apparent velocity is independent of whether the subject fixates on a stationary target or tracks the moving pattern. This is in contrast to egocentric motion perception in which the perceived velocity of the stimulus is greater by a factor of 1.6 when the eyes are kept stationary than when optokinetic nystagmus occurs (Dichgans et al., 1969). One may conclude

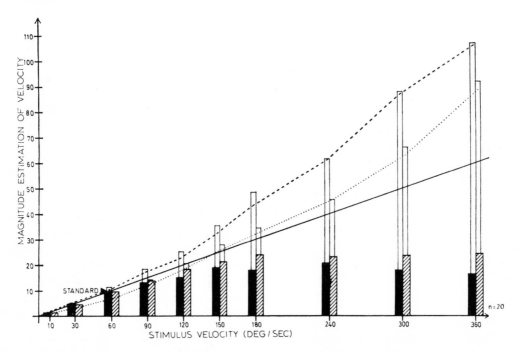

FIGURE 1 Magnitude estimations of velocity in egocentric (interrupted lines) and exocentric motion perception (dark columns). In each of these, velocities were scaled with fixation of a small stationary target (dashed line, black column) or with optokinetic nystagmus (dotted line, shaded column). The white columns symbolize estimates of apparent surround motion that with higher stimulus velocities occurs in addition to CV. The standard stimulus (modulus) is indicated by a black triangle. For further explanations see text.

that the visual motion information that leads to self-rotation sensation is abstracted before the differentiation between the two modes of egocentric velocity evaluation occurs.

With stimulus speeds exceeding 120°/sec, a mixed sensation occurs whereby the drum appears to rotate in the direction opposite to the perceived CV. The sum of the velocities of these apparent motions seems to correspond roughly to the phenomenal velocity of a stimulus that appears to move in reference to the stationary observer. The apparent velocity of CV moderately increases with stimulus speeds from 90° to 180°/sec and remains approximately constant with further increase of stimulus velocity up to the highest speeds tested (360°/sec).

Stimulus area and location within the visual field are the major factors in determining whether sensation of self-motion occurs or whether the stimulus is correctly perceived as moving relative to the observer. Experiments reported in detail by Brandt et al. (1973) showed that the peripheral retina dominates dynamic spatial orientation whereas the more central parts of the retina subserve egocentric motion perception, visual grasping, and eye tracking. As demonstrated in Figure 2, stimulation of the central parts of the visual field up to 30° in diameter scarcely ever leads to CV and even up to 60° yields only moderate CV. Moreover, central masking up to 120° in diameter has only a slightly diminishing effect on CV. The data in Figure 2 represent magnitude estimations of the subjective velocity of CV, but since both "intensity" and velocity strongly vary with each other, they are also representative for the rather ill-defined "compellingness" of the phenomenon. Obviously, an increase in the area stimulated by a moving pattern augments its effect on spatial orientation. But this is at least to a considerable extent due to the concurrent increase in the amount of peripheral retina included in stimulation. The predominating importance of the peripheral retina was further illustrated in an experiment where stimuli of equal area (30° in diameter) were exposed to the center and the periphery. It was evident that the peripheral stimuli yield stronger effects (Brandt et al., 1973).

In the experiment depicted in Figure 3, contradictory stimuli are applied that move in opposite directions across the center (30°) and the periphery of the visual field. In this case, exocentric and egocentric motion perception occur simultaneously. Again, the dynamic spatial orientation depends on the peripheral stimulus while the central stimulus is perceived as moving in reference to the observer. Optokinetic nystagmus subserving pattern perception is guided by the central stimulus despite its small area. The results not only illustrate the different functions of the center and periphery of the visual field but provide conclusive evidence that dynamic spatial orientation does not depend on the direction of eye movements.

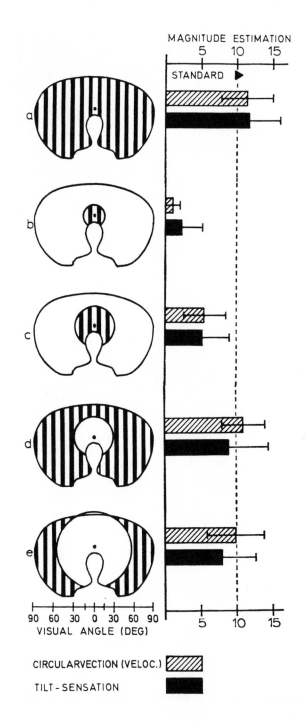

FIGURE 2 Magnitude estimates of subjective velocity (shaded columns) and tilt perceived during pseudo-Coriolis effects (black columns) in relation to variations of stimulus area and location within the visual field. Optokinetic stimuli (60°/sec) are schematically depicted on the left. Masks are symbolized by white areas. Particular importance of stimulation of the peripheral retina is shown in d and e in which central masks up to 120° in diameter (e) scarcely diminish CV and tilt. Stimulation of the more central retina yields rather small effects (b and c). Variations in perceived velocity and tilt sensation are strongly related to each other.

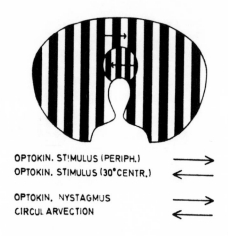

OPTOKIN. STIMULUS (PERIPH.)   ⟶
OPTOKIN. STIMULUS (30°CENTR.)   ⟵

OPTOKIN. NYSTAGMUS   ⟶
CIRCULARVECTION   ⟵

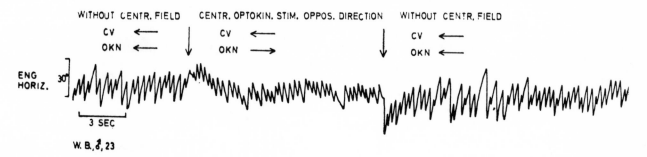

FIGURE 3   Opposite optokinetic stimulation of center and periphery. In this situation, CV is determined by the peripheral stimulus while optokinetic nystagmus (OKN) (lower graph) is guided by the central stimulus. As soon as the central stimulus appears, the direction of OKN reverses. The direction of CV is unaltered.

Moving visual scenes shift the apparent direction of gravity

Using visual displays without cues of visual orientation that could possibly conflict with cues of gravity, it has been demonstrated that seen motion as such may induce tilt of the apparent upright of visual contours and body posture (Dichgans et al., 1972). If a large visual display (130° of visual angle) is rotated around the observer's line of sight, a stationary central test edge, initially set to the vertical, seems to be tilted in the direction opposite to the rotation of the field. Subjects were asked to readjust continuously the orientation of the central test edge to vertical. The corrections made to compensate for perceived tilt were continuously recorded. The tilt illusion starts shortly after initiation of the movement, increases rapidly at first, then progressively more slowly, and reaches its steady state within an average of 18 sec. The amount of apparent tilt increases with angular velocity of the visual stimulus up to 30°/sec (Figure 4A). The estimated tilt averaged 15° for 7 subjects and exceeded 40° in one subject. In a second series of experiments on which we will extensively

report elsewhere (Held et al., in preparation), we found that tilt increases with stimulus area and that motion stimulation of the more peripheral parts of the retina exerts a disproportionately strong influence on the perceived upright (Figure 4B). This result corresponds with the observations on CV in which stimulation of the periphery dominates the induction of an apparent body motion. This latter stimulus condition also elicits the sensation of self-motion but, as described by Dichgans et al. (1972), the paradoxical sensation of continuous motion with limited tilt of the body occurs. The magnitude of tilt militates against the notion that small rotatory eye movements can account for the effect.

In order to demonstrate that the tilt effect is not an exclusively visual phenomenon but is due to a shift of the internal representation of the vector of gravity, we designed a second experiment in which tilt of the perceived postural upright was induced by motion stimulation. Subjects were seated in a moving-base airplane trainer (Link GAT 1). Using a control stick, they were able to adjust the position of the trainer to the subjective upright. A visual pattern was projected onto the side

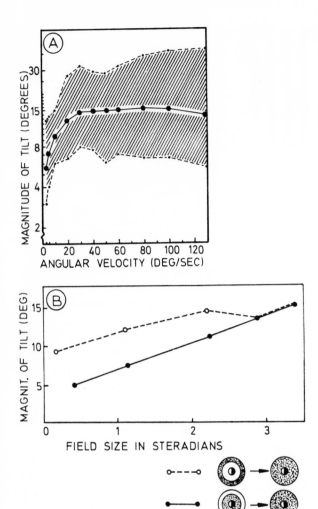

FIGURE 4 (A) Magnitude of apparent tilt of the visual vertical (geometric means on the solid line) in relation to velocity of the visual stimulus. The shaded region represents the range of single values of the 7 subjects. Interindividual data are highly replicable but individual variations are large. (B) Magnitude of apparent tilt in relation to stimulus area and location within the visual field (one subject). The size of the field was increased by either decreasing the outer radius or by increasing the inner radius of a white ring mask. Equal areas of stimulation (abscissa) yield greater tilt effects if exposed to the more peripheral parts of the visual field (open circles) than with stimulation of the more central retina (black dots).

windows of the trainer so as to move upward on one side and downward on the other. Shortly after the pattern was set into motion, the subjects started to roll the trainer's position off its initial vertical position. This was done in an attempt to compensate for the perceived tilt in postural orientation that, as in the case of the visual vertical, was opposite in direction to the moving stimulus. The resulting tilt of the cabin was therefore in the direction of the moving stimulus. It reached its steady stage after 17 sec and, with pattern velocities of 14 to 26°/sec, averaged 8.5° in 4 sub-

jects. The somewhat smaller effect on the perceived postural vertical may be due to the rather small area of motion stimulation and to graviceptive information originating from somatosensory pressure receptors that signal the induced change in body posture.

We have argued earlier that the tilt of both the visual and the postural vertical can be attributed to the visual motion stimulus alone (Dichgans et al., 1972). We have also stated that the perceptual effects are equivalent to the results of shifting the direction of gravity. Indeed, real displacement of the vector of gravity results in corresponding perceptions (Mach, 1875). This has been demonstrated in very thorough experiments by Clark and Graybiel (1951) and Graybiel (1952), who accomplished this effect in a human centrifuge. They found a "fairly good correspondence" between the subject's estimate of tilt in postural orientation and perceived visual vertical, on the one hand, and the angle between the direction of gravity and the vector of force resulting from gravity and centrifugal forces, on the other. We hypothesize that the orientation of the gravitational vector is computed by the central nervous system from graviceptive input originating in the labarynthine otoliths and somato sensory pressure receptors as well as from seen motion.

The possible neurophysiological mechanisms

Circularvection and the change in the apparent direction of gravity seem to be related phenomena: Both may be explained by the convergence of visual and vestibular information. So far, this possibility has only been examined in a few neurophysiological experiments in animals. Indeed, optokinetic stimulation can induce a direction-specific modulation of resting discharge in the vestibular nerve of the goldfish (Klinke and Schmidt, 1970) and the medial and lateral vestibular nuclei of the rabbit (Dichgans and Brandt, 1972). In the rabbit, some of the neurons in the vestibular nuclei respond not only to angular acceleration but also to exclusive visual motion stimulation without any head movement. The directional specificity of these neurons is opposite for visual and vestibular stimuli. This corresponds to the natural condition in which a rotation of the animal to the left is accompanied by relative motion of the environment to the right and vice versa. The prolonged summation and decay of frequency modulation after stimulus onset and termination roughly correspond to the time course of CV.

The anatomical pathways along which visual information is carried into the vestibular system are still to be investigated. Direct connections to the vestibular nuclei from either the lateral geniculate body or the superior colliculus are unknown. The long latencies for the induction of CV and apparent tilt of the vertical would suggest a multisynaptic pathway, possibly through the network of the reticular formation. The hypothesis that the superior colliculus would serve as an important relay within the circuit of convergence of visual information into the vertibular system for the purpose of dynamic spatial orientation seems to be attractive, for this structure reportedly represents a major center for visual and auditory orientation within a static environment. This notion, however, still lacks experimental evidence.

The preference of neurons in the superior colliculus for moving as opposed to stationary visual stimuli is evident in all mammalian species so far investigated. Sprague et al. (1973) pointed out that "it is only in the superior colliculus that movement is a specific trigger for the great majority of neurons," and he suggested "that behavioral performances involving detection of motion or rates of motion, are at least in part integrated by neuronal circuits taking an obligatory route through the superior colliculus."

At this point one should remember that the superior colliculus receives a clear-cut projection from the very peripheral retina (Apter, 1945; Forrester, 1967) whereas the projection to the lateral geniculate body originates mainly from the fovea and the more central parts of the retina (Bishop et al., 1962; recent review by Freund, 1973). It has been claimed that the superior colliculus of the monkey, in contrast to that of the cat, does not receive any direct projections from the fovea (Brouwer and Zeeman, 1926; Wilson and Toyne, 1970). Although still controversial, the latter finding would support the hypothesis of the superior colliculus being a major center for *ambient vision* and orientation (Trevarthen, 1968).

It has been indirectly shown by Klinke and Schmidt (1970) and Uemura and Cohen (1972) that the efferent vestibular pathway carries optokinetic information to the vestibular receptor. Nevertheless, numerous additional sites of visual-vestibular convergence are to be expected within the central nervous system.

The *functional importance* of visual motion information for the perception of self-motion may now be considered. With rotation or linear motion in a horizontal plane, the vestibular receptors signal only acceleration. Once constant velocity is reached, cupulae and otoliths slowly return to their resting position and the vestibular input dies out. Yet during constant velocity, even with passive movement, the perception of self-motion is maintained by visual motion information. This can easily be demonstrated. If, at constant velocity, one closes the eyes or if, in a rotating room, one is confronted with a seemingly stationary visual environment, motion is not perceived. With self-motion at constant velocity or at levels of acceleration below the vestibular threshold, visual input is obviously a most important source of information to

which kinesthesis may also contribute. The different functions of the peripheral retina and of its more central parts allow for adequate self-motion perception and for eye tracking and the perception of smaller objects moving in relation to the observer and his environment.

The functional importance of the second phenomenon in which the apparent direction of gravity is shifted by a visual stimulus moving in a vertical plane is not as well understood at the present time. It is generally accepted that "a coordinate system based on the direction of gravity forms the basis of a reference system by which man orients himself to the earth and to objects in space" (Graybiel, 1952). Since the internal estimate of the vector of gravity also depends on visual motion information, it is conceivable that the effect of relative motion of the visual surroundings caused by any body displacement from real upright would corroborate the actual information from gravireceptors for postural adjustment. Thus, the stability of visual and postural orientation with respect to gravity might depend in part upon motion within the observer's visual field. Visual stabilization of posture is evident in patients with a bilateral labyrynthine disease.

REFERENCES

APTER, J. T., 1945. The projection of the retina on superior colliculus of cats. *J. Neurophysiol.* 8:123–134.

BISHOP, P. O., W. KOZAK, W. R. LEVIK, and G. VAKKUR, 1962. The determination of the projection of the visual field onto the lateral geniculate nucleus of cat. *J. Physiol.* (*London*) 163:503–539.

BRANDT, TH., E. WIST, and J. DICHGANS, 1971. Optisch induzierte Pseudo-Coriolis-Effekte und Circularvektion: Ein Beitrag zur optisch-vestibulären Interaktion. *Arch. Psychiat. Nervenkr.* 214:365–389.

BRANDT, TH., J. DICHGANS, and E. KOENIG, 1973. Differential effects of central versus peripheral vision on egocentric and exocentric motion perception. *Exp. Brain Res.* (in press).

BROUWER, B., and W. P. C. ZEEMAN, 1926. The projection of the retina in the primary optic neurons in monkeys. *Brain* 49:1–35.

CLARK, B., and A. GRAYBIEL, 1951. Visual perception of the horizontal following exposure to radial acceleration on a centrifuge. *J. Comp. Physiol. Psychol.* 44:525–534.

DICHGANS, J., F. KÖRNER, and K. VOIGT, 1969. Vergleichende Skalierung des afferenten und efferenten Bewegungssehens beim Menschen: Lineare Funktionen mit verschiedener Anstiegssteilheit. *Psychol. Forsch.* 32:277–295.

DICHGANS, J., and TH. BRANDT, 1972. Visual-vestibular interaction and motion perception. In *Cerebral control of eye movements and motion perception*, J. Dichgans and E. Bizzi, eds. Basel and New York: S. Karger.

DICHGANS, J. R., R. HELD, L. R. YOUNG, and TH. BRANDT, 1972. Moving visual scenes influence the apparent direction of gravity. *Science* 178:1217–1219.

FISCHER, M. H., and A. E. KORNMÜLLER, 1930. Optokinetisch ausgelöste Bewegungswahrnehmungen und optokinetischer Nystagmus. *J. Psychol. Neurol.* (Lpz.) 41:273–308.

FORRESTER, J. M., and S. K. LAL, 1967. The projection of the rats visual field upon the superior colliculus. *J. Physiol. (London)* 189:25–26.

FREUND, H.-J., 1973. Neuronal mechanisms of the lateral geniculate body. In *Handbook of Sensory Physiology*, Vol. VII/3B, R. Jung, ed. Berlin, Heidelberg, New York: Springer-Verlag.

GRAYBIEL, A., 1952. Oculogravic illusion. *A.M.A. Arch. Ophthalmol.* 48:605–615.

GROEN, J. J., 1961. The problems of the spinning top applied to the semicircular canals. *Confin. Neurol. (Basel)* 21:454–455.

GURNEE, H., 1931. The effect of a visual stimulus upon the perception of bodily motion. *Amer. J. Psychol.* 43:26–48.

HELMHOLTZ, H. von, 1896. *Handbuch der physiologischen Optik*. Hamburg and Leipzig: Voss.

KLINKE, R., and C. L. SCHMIDT, 1970. Efferent influence on the vestibular organ during active movement of the body. *Pflügers Arch. ges. Physiol.* 318:325–332.

MACH, E., 1875. *Grundlinien der Lehre von den Bewegungsempfindungen*. Leipzig: Engelmann.

MACH, E., 1885. *Die Analyse der Empfindungen*. Jena: Fischer.

SPRAGUE, J. M., G. BERLUCCHI, and G. RIZZOLATTI, 1973. The role of the superior colliculus and pretectum in vision and visually guided behavior. In *Handbook of Sensory Physiology*, Vol. VII/3B, R. Jung, ed., Berlin, Heidelberg, New York: Springer.

TREVARTHEN, C. B., 1968. Two mechanisms of vision in primate. *Psychol. Forsch.* 31:229–337.

UEMURA, T., and B. COHEN, 1972. Vestibular-ocular reflexes: Effect of vestibular nuclei lesions. In *Progress in Brain Research, 37. Basic Aspects of Central Vestibular Mechanisms*. A. Brodal and O. Pompeiano, eds., Amsterdam: Elsevier.

WILSON, M. E., and M. J. TOYNE, 1970. Retino-tectal and corticotectal projections in Macaca Mulatta. *Brain Res.* 24:395–406.

WOOD, R. W., 1895. The "haunted swing" illusion. *Psychol. Rev.* 2:277–278.

YOUNG, L. R., J. DICHGANS, R. MURPHY, and TH. BRANDT, 1972. Influence of optokinetically induced self-rotation on perception of horizontal body acceleration. *Pflügers Arch.* 334 (Suppl. R): 78.

13 Neural Processes for the Detection of Acoustic Patterns and for Sound Localization

E. F. EVANS

ABSTRACT The processing of auditory stimulus information in the periphery of the auditory system rests largely on spectral analysis and the preservation of a certain amount of temporal information including that related to interaural differences. The auditory system appears to divide into two subsystems that can be differentiated anatomically and functionally, at the brainstem level at least, and that may be related to the processing of localization and pattern information, respectively. Central processing leads to a considerable complexity and diversity of neural response patterns and stimulus specificity. The latter manifests itself, particularly at the cortical level, as a preferential or specific selectivity for important temporal and spatial features of stimuli (including biologically significant sounds). There is some psychophysical, and considerable behavioral, evidence that such feature-sensitive neurons are required to abstract important features from a complex auditory environment.

Introduction

IN THIS BRIEF review, the emphasis and selection of material will be directed toward evidence for feature-sensitive mechanisms in the auditory nervous system. More comprehensive accounts of the neurophysiological data will be found elsewhere (e.g., Evans, 1971; Erulkar, 1972).

It is probably true that studies of the auditory system directed at this problem have not produced such coherent evidence for elements capable of feature detection as in the visual system. There are a number of identifiable reasons for this. First, there has been a preoccupation with the problem of pitch perception and its resolution in terms of rival *place* and *time* theories. There is now evidence that pitch perception itself may involve a type of central pattern recognition process (Houtsma and Goldstein, 1972; see Wilson, the following chapter). Then there is the difficulty that faces investigators wishing to use acoustic stimuli more complex than pure tones, of manip-

E. F. EVANS Medical Research Council Group in Neurophysiology, Department of Communication, University of Keele, Keele, Staffordshire, England

ulating and defining their parameters: For example, it is not possible to manipulate the temporal and frequency parameters of an acoustic stimulus completely independently. Figure 1 illustrates some of the stimuli that are used. Finally, there are important differences between the anatomical organization of the auditory and visual systems. Compared with the primary visual pathway—the retino-geniculo-striate pathway—impulses reach the auditory cortex by way of an indefinite number of synaptic interruptions (with four as a minimum, see Figure 3), and cross-connections. Hence the auditory cortex is more deleteriously affected by anaesthesia, particularly as far as neurons with feature-specific sensitivities are concerned.

Features of auditory stimuli

What constitutes a significant feature of a complex auditory stimulus is to a certain extent a matter of guesswork and intuition. A feature for one species may not be a feature for another. Thus, the relatively narrow band of supersonic energy in the bat vocalization is an extremely powerful stimulus feature for the noctuid moth (Roeder, 1971). Certain vocalizations of the squirrel monkey act as releasers of appropriate behavior patterns in that species alone (Winter et al., 1966).

Alternatively, a consideration of a stimulus itself may indicate distinctive features in the spectrum or wave form that we might expect to be significant (Figure 2). Thus, in many vocalizations, including human speech, several features are prominent, (Figure 2A), and indeed many have been shown to be important for speech perception (e.g., Liberman et al., 1959). Noise, of more or less limited bandwidth is the dominant component of certain consonants, transient bursts, or clicks. Frequency changes (Figures 1D and 1E) are characteristic of certain consonants and vowels, (such as the vowel "i" in Figure 2A). The relationship between the frequency components (formants) is another important feature of vowel sounds. Changes in amplitude (Figure 1B), or the envelope (as in

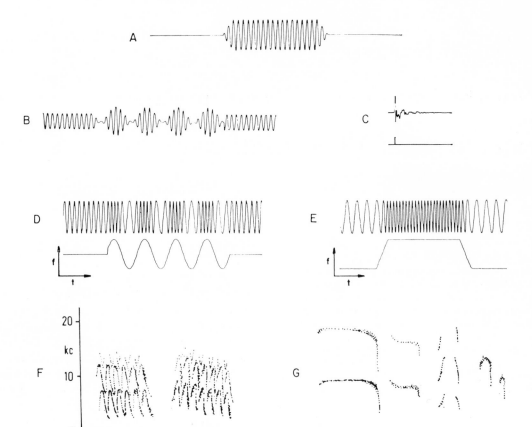

FIGURE 1 Simple and complex acoustic stimuli. A: Pure tone burst (onset and termination "shaped" to avoid click artifacts). B: Sinusoidally amplitude-modulated tone. C: Acoustic wave form of a "click" (upper trace) generated by a loudspeaker fed by an electrical pulse of short duration (lower trace). D: Sinusoidally frequency-modulated tone. Lower trace indicates excursions of frequency as a function of time. E: Linearly ("ramp") frequency-modulated tone. Lower trace as in D. F and G: Naturally occurring biologically significant stimuli; spectrograms of species-specific vocalizations of squirrel monkey. (From Winter et al., 1966.) F shows example of calls with approximately sinusoidal frequency modulation. G shows examples of calls with linear frequency modulation components.

Figure 2B) or "attack" of a sound can be distinctive features of sound complexes. The temporal patterning of the components of a stimulus can also be critical, as in the case of the distinctions between songs of different behavioral significance in the same species of cricket (Figure 2C). To this list of features should be added the dominant features for the localization of a sound source in space, namely, interaural differences in the time of arrival and the intensity of stimuli.

Alternatively, a number of acoustic features of complex sounds can be identified in that they are highly effective stimuli for neurons at the upper levels of the auditory system, as will be shown in a later section.

Two auditory systems for localization and form?

The complex anatomy of the auditory pathway may be made more comprehensible by recent evidence supporting a division of the lower levels by the older anatomists (Poljak, 1926) into two separable subsystems (Figure 3). On anatomical grounds, Poljak suggested that the ventral pathway originating in the ventral cochlear nucleus and including the trapezoid body and superior olivary nuclei might subserve localization and reflex functions, whereas the dorsal pathway might subserve discriminatory function.

These two pathways first separate in the cochlear nucleus, in the ventral and dorsal divisions, respectively. Early experiments recording single unit activity in the cochlear nucleus (e.g., Rose et al., 1959) did not find significant differences between the morphologically very different ventral and dorsal nuclei. However, data obtained in the unanaesthetized cat (Evans and Nelson, 1973a) and in other preparations (reviewed in Evans and Nelson, 1973a) indicate that they are substantially different in their functional properties.

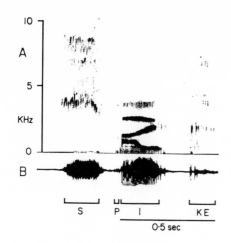

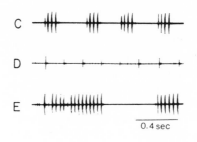

FIGURE 2 Features of naturally occurring acoustic stimuli. A and B: Human speech, illustrated by the utterance "SPIKE." A: Spectrogram. Note broad-band but differing distributions of energy in the "S," "P," and "KE" regions; multiple frequency components (formants) of the vowel "I" and the frequency transitions of the lowest two formants; the click-like transient at onset of K. B: Wave form. C, D, and E: Three types of songs in male crickets. C: Calling. D: Courtship. E: Rivalry song. (From Huber, 1972.)

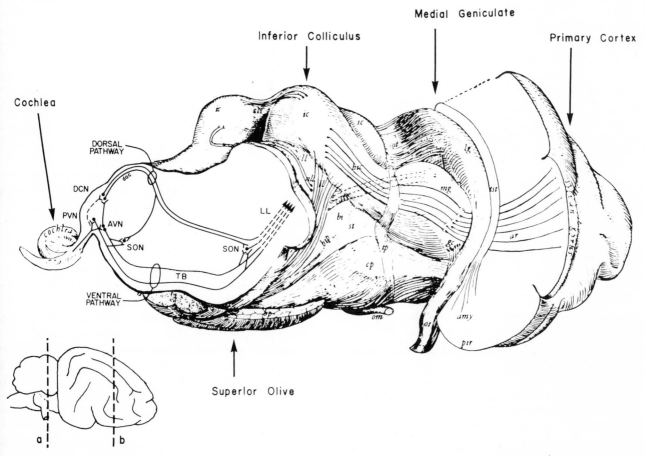

FIGURE 3 Simplified diagram of auditory pathways in cat. The brain has been sectioned across the brainstem (section a of inset), and the cerebellum and cerebral cortex removed up to incision b. The pathway consists, as a minimum, of the following steps: cochlear nerve; dorsal pathway via dorsal cochlear nucleus (DCN) to lateral lemniscus (LL); ventral pathway via anterior (AVN) and posterior (PVN) ventral cochlear nucleus subdivisions, trapezoid body (TB) and superior olivary nuclei (SON); lateral lemniscus (LL); inferior colliculus (ic); medial geniculate nucleus (mg); primary projection cortex; secondary areas (not shown). (After Papez, 1967, and Evans and Nelson, 1973b.)

To a first approximation, the responses of the *ventral pathway* reflect the properties of primary auditory neurons. An increase in firing rate (excitation) of short latency and with relatively little adaptation during sustained stimulation (Figure 4A) is characteristic of the responses of most neurons in the ventral cochlear nucleus (e.g., Rose et al., 1959; Evans and Nelson, 1973a) and superior olive (e.g., Tsuchitani and Boudreau, 1966). The responses occur over a restricted range of frequencies comparable to those of fibers in the cochlear nerve. Primary auditory neurons have a high degree of frequency

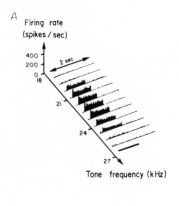

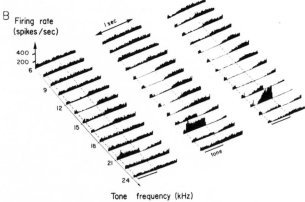

FIGURE 4   Ventral and dorsal pathway responses. A: Response characteristic of neurons in ventral pathway. Array of histograms of activity before, during and after 1 sec tone (indicated by bar), taken at the tonal frequencies indicated, at 15 dB above threshold. Each histogram represents the average of 7 tone presentations. Note that the only response is sustained excitation across the response band. B: Response characteristic of many neurons in dorsal pathway. Array of time histograms as in A, at three intensity levels: 10, 20, and 30 dB above threshold, respectively, from left to right. Each histogram represents the average of 10 tone presentations. Note extensive frequency band of inhibition sustained throughout and following the tone (indicated by bar and interrupted lines), particularly at higher intensities; small "island" of excitation arising from "sea" of inhibition, with complex time course, indicating delayed inhibition. Dorsal cochlear nucleus under chloralose. (After Evans and Nelson, 1973a.)

selectivity (Kiang et al., 1965, 1967; Evans, 1972), and this is retained for signals of greater complexity than pure tones (de Boer, 1969; Evans and Wilson, 1971; Wilson and Evans, 1971). This selectivity is approximately equivalent to that of the filters responsible for the spectrograms of Figures 1F, 1G, and 2A. The neurons of the ventral pathway are furthermore tightly organized on the basis of their optimum frequency sensitivity (*characteristic* or *best* frequency), that is, the pathway is tonotopically organized (Rose et al., 1959; Evans and Nelson, 1973a), and this is preserved in the superior olive (Tsuchitani and Boudreau, 1966). Hence, the distribution of neural activity across the ventral pathway in response to a complex signal will at least, to a first approximation, resemble a typical spectrographic analysis of that signal.

The ventral pathway also preserves a certain amount of temporal information. The spike discharges of many (but not all, see Rupert and Moushegian, 1970) neurons are time locked to a particular phase of the stimulus, for frequencies below about 4 to 5 kHz, and at least at the cochlear nerve level can more or less faithfully reproduce a rectified version of the wave form of complex low-frequency stimuli (reviewed by Hind, 1972). It is not by any means certain that the auditory system can make use of this temporal information for the analysis of simple and complex acoustic patterns (see Houtsma and Goldstein, 1972; Goldstein, 1972), but preservation of time information is necessary for the analysis by the superior olive of the differences in times of arrival of signals at the two ears, as is shown in the next section.

The *dorsal pathway* arises in the morphologically complex dorsal division of the cochlear nucleus, receiving its input at least in part by way of intranuclear connections from the ventral division (Evans and Nelson, 1968, 1973b). A wide variety of responses to tones can be obtained in the dorsal cochlear nucleus, particularly in the unanaesthetized preparation, analogous to those of retinal ganglion cells (especially the *Y*-cells: See Wright earlier in this part). Some neurons give excitatory responses to tones over a restricted range of frequencies and are inhibited by contiguous frequency bands of considerable extent (Figure 4B). Others exhibit only inhibitory responses to tones. The time course of the response can be a very complex sequence of excitation and inhibition (including "after discharges") dependent upon the stimulus frequency, and intensity (Figure 4B), and repetition rate.

The ventral and dorsal pathways converge in the lateral lemnisci. Whether they retain their separate identities at the higher levels of the auditory pathway remains to be shown; however, the responses of neurons in the inferior colliculi (e.g., Rose et al., 1963), medial geniculate nuclei (e.g., Adrian et al., 1966) and auditory cortex (e.g., Bogdanski and Galambos, 1960; Katsuki et al., 1962; Evans and Whitfield, 1964; Goldstein et al., 1968) show great variety and complexity compared with those of the lower levels, particularly of the ventral pathway.

This division of the ascending auditory system into two anatomically and functionally separable subsystems may turn out to be analogous to the two major subsystems proposed for the visual system (e.g., by Held et al., 1967) subserving, respectively, the processing of place and form information.

Neural analysis of cues for sound location

Information in the ventral pathways from the two ears first converges in the superior olive, particularly in the accessory nucleus. The cells of the latter have two transverse dendrites that, respectively, receive input from each ear (Moushegian et al., 1964; Hall, 1965).

Hall (1965) described a number of types of response in the accessory nucleus of the cat, which were determined by excitatory input from the contralateral, and inhibitory input from the ipsilateral, ear. Of most interest, were responses from what he called "time-intensity trading" cells (Figure 5). The probability of discharge is related to both the interaural time delay and the interaural intensity differences of the signal in such a way that the effects of one can be traded against the other to maintain a constant level of response. Thus, to maintain the probability of discharge in the neuron of Figure 5 at a level corresponding to zero interaural delay at equal signal levels to both ears (i.e., ca. 0.1) when the level at the left ear is reduced by 10 dB (middle curve), requires the signal to the left ear to be advanced relative to the right ear by about

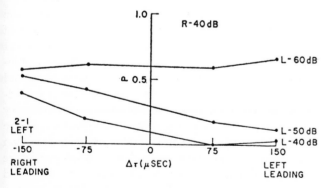

FIGURE 5 "Time-intensity trading" in a neuron in the accessory nucleus of the cat superior olive (see text). *Ordinate*: Probability of discharge of neuron in response to a click stimulus presented to each ear with the interaural delay indicated by the abscissa. Intensity at right ear constant at 40 dB below a reference level; to the left ear 40, 50, and 60 dB below the reference level, as indicated to the right of the respective plots. (From Hall, 1965.)

150 μsec (i.e., right-most point of middle curve). Hall has shown that the extent of this "time-intensity trading" is of the same order of magnitude as that observed psychophysically in man.

At the inferior colliculus level (again in the cat), Rose et al. (1966) have demonstrated that for some neurons of low (less than 3 kHz) characteristic frequency, their discharge is dependent upon the interaural time delay but is independent within wide limits of frequency and absolute intensity (Figure 6). The probability of discharge reaches a maximum at a so-called "critical delay" (140 μsec in the example of Figure 6) virtually irrespective of the stimulus frequency and of the stimulus intensity (over 60 dB in one unit). The "critical delay neuron" of Figure 6 could serve to signal sound source locations about 35° from the midline sagittal plane of the cat's head. The importance of this exciting observation has been called into question by Moushegian, Stillman, and Rupert (1972) on two grounds. First, they found "critical delays" in the inferior colliculus of the kangaroo cat restricted to interaural delays of 100 to 300 μsec. Compared with the maximum naturally occurring interaural stimulus delay in this species of 105 μsec, these "critical delays" are unlikely to be of behavioral significance for localization of the sound source. Second, they pointed out that the "critical delays" are not critical, that is, they represent a broad peak or plateau of discharge rate over a range of the order of 100 μsec, which is large compared with the maximum interaural delay, even in the cat (ca. 250 μsec).

Also in the inferior colliculus, Rose et al. (1966) found a few neurons of low and high characteristic frequencies that were exquisitely sensitive to very small binaural intensity differences (of a few dB). This sensitivity persisted over a wide range of absolute levels of the binaural stimuli. Such neurons would be important for the localization of continuous sounds of frequency in excess of that at which timing mechanisms would cease to operate.

Geisler et al. (1969) have shown that the above observations also obtain for wide-band noise stimuli.

A further level of processing appears to obtain in the cat inferior colliculus. Altman (1968) discovered neurons that were sensitive to the virtual *direction of movement* of a train of click stimuli. For these neurons to respond, virtual sound sources on one side of the head or in a small segment of space had to move in a certain direction, i.e., toward or away from the midline.

Comparing responses at both the collicular and superior olivary levels, Altman (1971) has concluded that collicular neurons demonstrate a higher degree of specificity to particular ranges of interaural time or intensity differences approaching an order of magnitude, in terms of change in impulse discharge rate, for equal changes in stimulus parameters.

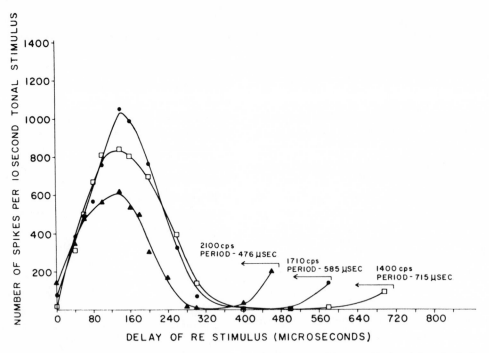

FIGURE 6 "Critical delay" neuron in inferior colliculus of cat. *Ordinate*: Number of spikes evoked by a 10 sec tone of the frequencies indicated as the parameters, presented to the two ears, the right ear (RE) signal being delayed relative to the left by the time indicated on the abscissa. (From Rose et al., 1966.)

Similar sensitivities to stimulus parameters related to the location of the sound source are shown by cortical neurons (Evans, 1968; Hall and Goldstein, 1968; Brugge et al., 1969). In a study in the unanaesthetized unrestrained cat, Evans (1968) found that 56% of the neurons in the primary cortices showed some preference for a certain location, and 31% *required* a certain location for any response. The majority required or preferred a contralateral location. A smaller number (9% and 4%, respectively) preferred or required an ipsilateral location for response. A few units responded only when the sound source was situated in the median sagittal plane anterior to the cat's head. Locations more than a few degrees on either side of this plane were ineffective. About 10% of the units were responsive to stimuli originating within the visual fields, and most of these responded only when the animal was both observing and listening to the sound source. Thus, the neurons that Hubel et al. (1969) described as "attention units" may merely represent neurons requiring simultaneous visual and auditory stimulation and having superimposable visual and auditory spatial receptive fields. It is apparent from the "case histories" of Hubel's unit that the criterion for "attention" was that the animal turned to look at the stimulus. The bimodally sensitive units appear to be analogous to those described by Spinelli et al. (1968) and Morrell (1972) in the visual cortex of the cat. Wickelgren (1971) has described similar neurons in the cat superior colliculus that had the ad-

ditional property of sensitivity to movement of the sound source.

Neural analysis of acoustic features

Probably the first evidence suggesting that the auditory system contained neural mechanisms sensitive to particular features of complex auditory stimuli came from an analysis of neurons in the primary auditory cortex of the unanaesthetized unrestrained cat by Bogdanski and Galambos (1960). Evans and Whitfield (1964; Whitfield and Evans, 1965; summarized in Evans, 1968), using the same preparation, Katsuki et al. (1962) in the monkey, Suga (e.g., 1965, 1972) in the anaesthetized bat, and Goldstein et al. (1968) using the unanaesthetized paralyzed cat preparation, have obtained similar but more comprehensive data.

Cortical neurons recorded under these conditions show striking differences from neurons at the lower levels of the auditory system discussed above. Thus, auditory cortical neurons exhibit a wide variety of stimulus sensitivities and response forms (Table I allows a comparison of results from a number of studies). In the first place, not all auditory cortical neurons respond to tonal stimuli. In the complete study of Evans and Whitfield, (Evans, 1965, 1968), less than three-quarters of the neurons responded to tones and many of these not consistently, unless certain manipulations of the spatial and temporal parameters of

TABLE I

Percentages of neurons with the characteristics indicated found in primary auditory cortex by various authors

Neurons in A1	Authors*				
	A (%)	B (%)	C (%)	D (%)	E (%)
1. Responding to sound	82	85–95	98		
2. Responding to tonal stimuli	70	57–77	82		
3. Not responding to tones but to some sound complex	12	21–18	16		
4. Responding to white noise	66		65		
5. Responding only to white noise			3.5		
6. Responding to click stimuli	26		52		
7. Responding only to click stimuli			1.5		
8. Not responding to steady tones but to frequency modulation		6–5		13	14

*A: Bogdanski and Galambos (1960), unanaesthetized unrestrained cat. B: Evans and Whitfield (Evans, 1965), unanaesthetized unrestrained cat. The first and second figures in the ranges given indicate respectively: the mean for all experiments and the figures obtained in the later experiments of the series where recording technique had been improved and where the location of the sound source in space was adjusted to give optimal responses. C: Goldstein, Hall, and Butterfield (1968), unanaesthetized paralysed cat. Each neuron was tested with stimuli presented binaurally and separately to each ear. D: Vardapetyan (1967), cat anaesthetized with chloralose. E: Suga (1965), bat anaesthetized with pentobarbitone. Includes unspecified number of neurons responding to steady tones but having pure tone thresholds more than 10 dB above those to frequency-modulated tones.

the stimuli were made. About 3% of the neurons responded only to a visual stimulus, generally movement of an edge. A further group of neurons (see the previous section) responded to both visual and auditory stimuli. About one-fifth of the population could not be driven by tonal stimuli but by complex sounds such as clicks, noise, and "kissing" sounds—that is, the "back-door" noises used for human communication with pet felines! Those neurons that did respond to tones did so in a variety of ways depending upon the neuron, and often upon the frequency and intensity of the tonal stimuli. These responses comprise sustained excitation, inhibition, and transient responses at the onset, termination, and onset and termination of the pure tones. About 5% of the total population (about 10% of the neurons responding to tones) responded only if the frequency was changing. The frequency selectivity of many cortical neurons is wide or indeterminate (Katsuki et al., 1959; Evans and

Whitfield, 1964), compared with the well-defined and restricted frequency selectivity at the level of the cochlear nerve (Kiang et al., 1965; Evans, 1972).

Many cortical neurons, then, at least in unanaesthetized preparations, appear to be less "interested" in the classically studied parameters of acoustic stimuli, namely, the frequency and intensity of continuous tones, than in certain less easily definable features of complex sounds. A considerable body of data has been collected, notably by Suga (in the bat: summarized, 1972), on the responses of neurons at the upper levels of the auditory system to noise, frequency- and amplitude-modulated stimuli, and to stimuli patterned in frequency and in time.

NOISE   The above-mentioned studies by Bogdanski and Galambos (1960), Evans and Whitfield (1964), and Goldstein et al. (1968) indicated that broadband stimuli (such as rattling keys, kissing noises, etc.) were extremely effective for many cortical neurons in the cat, in the sense that these stimuli gave responses more consistently or at lower thresholds than did pure tones. Up to 20% of cortical neurons could be driven *only* by noise complexes. (Smaller percentages are recorded when unstructured white noise stimuli are used; Table I.) Such "noise-specialized" neurons have been described in the inferior colliculus and cortex of the anaesthetized bat (Suga, 1972). At the periphery, neurons respond to noise stimuli as if the latter were filtered in accordance with their frequency-threshold "tuning" curves, and consequently the noise threshold is always 10 to 20 dB *higher* than that of pure tones (Evans and Wilson, 1971; Moller, 1970). That the reverse is the case in these cortical neurons must presumably arise from central convergence of spectral information in the manner of a logical AND operation: The need for activation of a number of spectrally separate inputs would increase the tone threshold relative to that for noise.

FREQUENCY MODULATION   Bogdanski and Galambos (1960) were the first to report the presence, in the auditory cortex of unanaesthetized cats, of neurons specifically sensitive to changes in the frequency of tones but which were unstimulable by steady tones. Independently, Evans and Whitfield (1964), in the cat cortex, and Suga (1964, 1965), in the inferior colliculus and cortex of the bat, observed similar neurons and subjected them to more detailed study (Whitfield and Evans, 1965). Many of the findings have been confirmed by Vardapetyan (1967) and by Goldstein et al. (1968) in the cat auditory cortex.

While many cortical neurons gave more consistent responses to frequency-modulated tones than to steady tones, in the study of Evans and Whitfield (1964) 10% of the units responding to tones did so *only* if the frequency was changing. Goldstein et al. (1968) found such neurons to be "in the minority." Vardapetyan (1967) and Suga

(1965) encountered such "FM specialized" properties in nearly one-eighth of the neurons in their studies of the anaesthetized cat and bat, respectively.

For these neurons preferentially or specifically sensitive to frequency change, the direction and the rate of change are important parameters. Thus some will respond only to frequency changes in an upward (low- to high-frequency) direction, others to downward frequency changes, and others to both directions of change. With sinusoidal modulation of frequency, these neurons respond to more or less restricted regions of modulation rates within the range 0.5 to 15 cycle/sec (Whitfield and Evans, 1965; see also Figure 7A; Evans and Jolley, unpublished data). This selectivity for modulation rate may relate to the recent psychophysical evidence for frequency modulation sensitive "channels" in the human auditory system of Kay and Matthews (1971, 1972; see also Figure 7B). These channels can be adapted by pre-exposure to a tone frequency modulated at a given rate so that the detection threshold for stimuli modulated at that rate is raised by as much as a factor of 3, whereas the threshold to neighboring rates is less affected. As far as the neurons are concerned, the upper limit of the range of effective sinusoidal modulation rates appears to be determined more by the rate of *repetition* of the frequency change rather than the rate of change *per se*. The use of intermittent linear ramps of

frequency change indicates that cortical units can respond to almost instantaneous changes in frequency (Whitfield and Evans, 1965).

Neurons sensitive to the direction of frequency change have been found in smaller numbers at lower levels of the auditory pathway: in the inferior colliculus (Suga, 1964, 1965; Nelson et al., 1966; Vartanian, 1971), in the superior olivary nucleus (Watenabe and Ohgushi, 1968), and to a much lesser extent in the cochlear nucleus (Evans and Nelson, 1966a, 1966b; Erulkar et al., 1968). However, neurons responding specifically (that is, *only*) to frequency-modulated tones have not been reported at levels lower than the inferior colliculus. Suga (1968, 1972) has made a detailed study of these neurons at this level in the bat and describes an additional selectivity, namely for the *form* of the frequency sweep (e.g., linear or exponential).

AMPLITUDE MODULATION   Nelson et al. (1966) found a number of neurons in the inferior colliculus of the anaesthetized cat that exhibited some selectivity to tonal stimuli sinusoidally modulated in amplitude. Some neurons would respond *only* to amplitude-modulated stimuli. Many were sensitive to the direction of modulation. In these cases, the nature and magnitude of the responses were critically dependent upon the rate and depth of modulation.

A

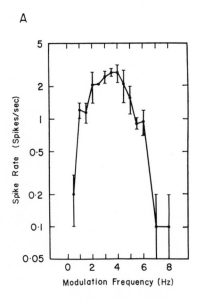

B

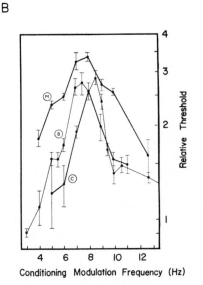

FIGURE 7   Selectivity of cat auditory cortical neurons and human auditory system for rate of frequency modulation. A: Mean spike rate (and range) of neuron in cat primary auditory cortex in response to tone at characteristic frequency modulated sinusoidally at rate indicated on abscissa. (Evans and Jolley, unpublished observations.) B: Psychophysical selectivity to sinusoidal frequency modulation. *Ordinate*: Elevation of detection threshold for frequency modulation of 250 Hz tone mod-

ulated at 8 Hz, after exposure to same tone modulated at the rates indicated on the abscissa. (Conditioning and test tones at 40 to 45 dB above pure tone threshold). M, B, and C: monaural, binaural and contra-aural testing, respectively, of three subjects; bars indicate 95% confidence limits. (After Kay and Matthews, 1971.) While the relationship between the ordinate scales of A and B is arbitrary, it is nevertheless apparent that the modulation frequencies and selectivities are comparable.

Vartanyan (1970) has confirmed these findings in the inferior colliculus of the anaesthetized rat. Selectivity was limited to a few neurons of the class that exhibited transient onset responses to tones. These neurons responded either by reproducing the modulation rhythm or by an increase in their mean discharge rate to stimuli modulated within a relatively restricted range of rates occurring above 10 cycle/sec. Thus, they illustrate a neuron that responded to modulation rates only within the range 20 to 30 cycle/sec. By contrast, neurons that gave sustained responses to tonal stimuli reproduced the modulation rhythm over a wide range of modulation rates, with little evidence of selectivity within ranges of 5 to 100 cycle/sec, in some cases.

Vartanyan (1971) has studied the thresholds of collicular neurons also as a function of the rise time of tonal stimuli. Whereas those for neurons responding in a sustained manner to tones were invariant for rise times up to as long as 70 msec, the thresholds for neurons responding transiently to tones were substantially greater for rise times above 5 msec.

In the inferior colliculus of the bat, Suga (1971) found responses dependent upon the rise time of noise and tone stimuli. In particular, some neurons had an "upper threshold" above which sounds failed to excite, determined by the rate and extent of the rise of the amplitude envelope. Below certain rates of rise, the upper threshold was absent. In other neurons, variations in rise time produced systematic changes in the sizes of the frequency threshold response areas: For some, increasing the rise time increased the extent; for other neurons, the response area was reduced. Suga considered these neurons to be specialized for responding to particular rise times. On the other hand, 26% of his sample had latency and response patterns that were not affected over a wide range of stimulus amplitudes and rise times.

More recently, Swarbrick and Whitfield (1972) described a few neurons in the primary auditory cortex of the unanaesthetized cat that appeared to be sensitive to the degree of symmetry of the amplitude envelope of noise bursts. Some neurons responded maximally to symmetrical envelopes, others to asymmetrical envelopes (e.g., where the rise versus fall time was less than 1:5), both types being independent of the duration of the stimulus over a tenfold range. These neurons appear to be selectively responsive to the "shape" of acoustic stimuli.

MULTIPLE FREQUENCY PATTERNS There are relatively few reports of systematic studies of the responses of neurons to stimuli composed of more than one frequency component. Multicomponent stimuli (i.e., comb-filtered noise) have been utilized for examining the frequency resolving power of primary auditory neurons (Evans et al.,

1971; Wilson and Evans, 1971). At this level a straightforward spectral analysis appears to take place: The neurons respond as would be predicted on the basis that their pure tone frequency threshold characteristics represent linear (one-half to one-tenth octave) filtering.

Oonishi and Katsuki (1965) found neurons in the auditory cortex of the lightly anaesthetized cat that exhibited peaks of sensitivity at more than one band of frequencies. The most common frequency ratio between the peaks was 2:1 or 2.5:1. Abeles and Goldstein (1972) and Evans and Jolley (unpublished results) have observed similar multipeak frequency response areas in cortical neurons of unanaesthetized and lightly anaesthetized preparations, respectively.

Oonishi and Katsuki (1965) and Abeles and Goldstein (1972) subjected the cortical neurons under their study to two-component tonal stimuli. They observed various patterns of facilitation and inhibition, depending upon the frequency separation of the tones and the nature of the neurons' response area. Whereas the former authors encountered unexpected sensitivities to two simultaneous tones, Abeles and Goldstein were unable to find evidence of neurons with response magnitudes to two tone stimuli that could not be attained by single tones.

Feher and Whitfield (1966) attempted to drive, by combinations of stimuli, the significant proportion of neurons that in the unanaesthetized cat could not be stimulated by single tonal stimuli. They succeeded in producing responses in a few such neurons with a combination of a pure and a frequency-modulated tone. The effective combination was fairly specific: Similar differences of frequency in adjacent portions of the spectrum were ineffective.

TEMPORAL PATTERNING It has already been mentioned that many of the neurons recorded from the auditory cortex of the unanaesthetized cat give labile responses to tonal stimuli unless manipulations are made of certain stimulus parameters. One of these parameters is the temporal patterning of the tones independent of any changes in frequency (Figure 8; Evans, 1968). The responses to tones of most cortical neurons in this preparation habituate rapidly (Figure 8A). By contrast, a few neurons require repeated presentations of the same stimulus for response (Figure 8B). Most cortical neurons exhibiting responses to the termination of tones ("off" responses) responded more vigorously to tones of longer duration than to short tones (Figures 8C, 8D); in a few others only short duration tones evoked consistent responses (Figure 8E).

The temporal patterning of component "chirps" is an essential feature distinguishing various calls of the cricket (Figures 3C to 3E). Huber and his colleagues (see Huber,

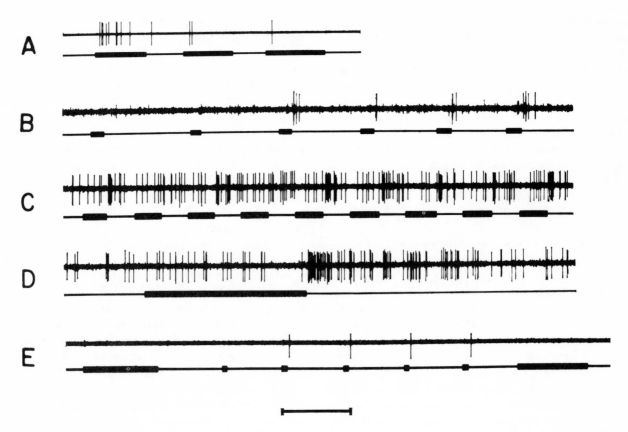

FIGURE 8   Sensitivity of auditory cortical neurons for temporal pattern. Neurons in AI of unanaesthetized cat. A: Rapid habituation of response to the repetitive presentation of a tone (at characteristic frequency of neuron). B: "Off" response re- quiring frequent repetitions of the same tone. C and D: Typical "off" response of a neuron; more vigorous response to tones of longer duration. E: "Off" response of a neuron to tones of short duration only. Time bar: 1 sec. (From Evans, 1968.)

1972) have identified two classes of interneurons in female crickets (*Gryllus*), one selective to the rate of occurrence and the duration of each chirp, and the other to the sequence of pulse components of individual chirps. With these interneurons, it is suggested that the female is able to distinguish the species-specific calls.

Neural analysis of biologically significant sound patterns

One of the first attempts to investigate the neural mech-anisms underlying an organisms' sensitivity to meaningful or significant sounds, was that of Frishkopf et al. (1966, 1968). They observed that the mating call of mature male North American bullfrogs (*Rana catesbeiana*) consisted of two main spectral components with peak energies at 0.3 and 1.5 kHz. These frequencies corresponded to the characteristic frequencies of two groups of neurons found in the bullfrog's auditory nerve, arising from the amphib-ian and basilar papillae, respectively. Synthetic calls comprising two peaks of energy and even two tone

stimuli at these frequencies evoked behavioral responses, i.e., responsive calling in other males. Since calls contain-ing only one peak of energy (i.e., at a single frequency) were behaviorally ineffective, Frishkopf and his col-leagues searched for neurons in the bullfrog's medulla and midbrain that were sensitive to the simultaneous presence of energy in the two frequency bands—a "mating call detector." Their search was unsuccessful. Related studies on the cricket frog (*Acris crepitans*; see Capranica and Frishkopf, 1972 for, review) however, indicated that the characteristic frequencies of auditory neurons in the medulla corresponded to the frequency spectrum of the call of male cricket frogs from that geographical region.

Konishi (1970) has assembled much evidence from studies of various birds to indicate that the spectral sensi-tivities of neurons at the medullary levels of the auditory system "match" to a greater or lesser extent the spectral energy distribution of the bird's own song. In particular, there is excellent correspondence between the upper limits of the neural and vocal frequency distributions.

Undoubtedly the most exciting work in this direction has been that on the squirrel monkey (*Saimiri sciureus*) by the late P. Winter in collaboration with Funkenstein and Nelson (1970, 1971, 1972) and their successors in Nelson's laboratory, Wollberg and Newman (1972). This monkey is found in the dense arboreal regions of South America and has a highly developed repertoire of vocalizations of social significance. Some 20 to 30 of these vocalizations have been spectrographically and behaviorally characterized in Ploog's laboratory in Munich (Winter et al., 1966). At least five main groups of calls have been established: "Distancing" calls emitted for example during feeding (see Figure 1F), acoustical contact calls (see Figure 1G), and calls related to directed aggression, to general aggression, and to high excitement. These calls consist of patterns of formants with characteristic frequencies and transitions (frequency modulation). Winter and his colleagues (Funkenstein et al., 1970; Winter and Funkenstein, 1971; Winter, 1972) demonstrated that many of the neurons in the primary auditory cortex of unanaesthetized squirrel monkeys were sensitive to certain of the vocalizations. Of 283 neurons tested, 41% responded to vocalizations and tonal as well as noise stimuli. Ten percent responded differentially between the natural and laboratory stimuli. Of these, 3.5% were selective for the vocalizations; that is, they did not respond to the laboratory stimuli tried. The selectivity was limited to one specific call type or calls with very similar acoustic properties (Figure 9A). It is noteworthy that in the example of Figure 9A, the discharges of the three neurons illustrated do not commence until as much as 200 msec after the onset of the nearly sinusoidal frequency modulation characteristic of the "trill" call. Wollberg and Newman (1972) have confirmed these important findings. Figure 9B illustrates a neuron from their study that did not respond to pure tones (note absence of response in the frequency array of dot displays in Figure 9F) but that was excited by calls from the "isolation peep" (acoustic contact) (plot B) and not by others (plots C to E; G to J).

Feature sensitive neurons and feature extraction

Sufficient evidence has been adduced above to indicate that a significant proportion of neurons in the upper levels of the auditory system are specifically or preferentially sensitive to certain features of complex auditory stimuli. The question arises whether these neurons subserve the function of feature detectors or extractors in the nervous system.

In the case of the acoustic neurons responsible for the detection of the presence of insectivorous bats, in the noctuid moth (reviewed in Roeder, 1971), the feature detection properties are obvious. It is debatable, however, whether many of the neurons whose properties have been

outlined above can justifiably be termed feature detectors. For the present it seems wise to reserve judgment and to use the operational term "feature sensitive."

Against an optimistic interpretation of the role of these neurons, it must be recognized that investigations involving recordings from single neurons at upper levels of the auditory system in unanaesthetized animals cannot entirely exclude or control other factors besides the "specific" stimulus features under study. Stimuli (particularly natural vocalizations) that evoke greater or lesser modifications of the state of "arousal" or "attention" of the animal may produce responses that, though appearing to be specific, are in fact not. Here, however, we appear to be faced with a paradox. Given that certain stimuli do evoke behavioral (e.g., "attention") responses, how can the investigator on the one hand completely exclude nonspecific effects on the cells under study, or on the other hand exclude that cell from the neural apparatus responsible in the first place for the modification in the animal's attention? Yet another difficulty arises from the recent report that the inconsistent responses given to steady tonal stimuli by cortical neurons in the unanaesthetized animal may become consistent if the animal is trained to respond to tonal stimuli, irrespective of whether the animal is actually responding at the time (Miller et al., 1972).

Against such objections, it is clear that many of the feature sensitivities reported above can be found (albeit in smaller numbers) in anaesthetized animals irrespective of the state of arousal. Furthermore, in unanaesthetized animals, in the case of the neurons specifically selective for one stimulus (e.g., one out of a number of species-specific vocalizations), stimuli that could be expected to evoke similar behavioral responses are ineffective, or produce inhibitory response (Figure 9B, plots B, C, E, and H).

Certainly, the neurons described in this chapter are endowed with properties that could be of analytical value to an organism. Specifically, cortical neurons are capable of providing "answers" to the following questions: Is the stimulus a noise, a click, a tone, or a species-specific call? Is the stimulus on? Has it just commenced? Has it just been terminated? What is its duration and its repetition rate? Is the frequency changing? If so, in which direction, at what rate? How rapidly is the amplitude rising? Where is the stimulus located in space? Is it moving? And so on. On the other hand, stimulus parameters such as frequency and intensity *per se* are not well represented in the responses of many cortical cells. There is a large body of data that suggests that it is the potentially abstractive functions that are preferentially lost in cases of cortical damage.

Ablation of the auditory cortex has been shown to interfere severely with the ability of animals (cat and monkey) to make discriminations based on the duration,

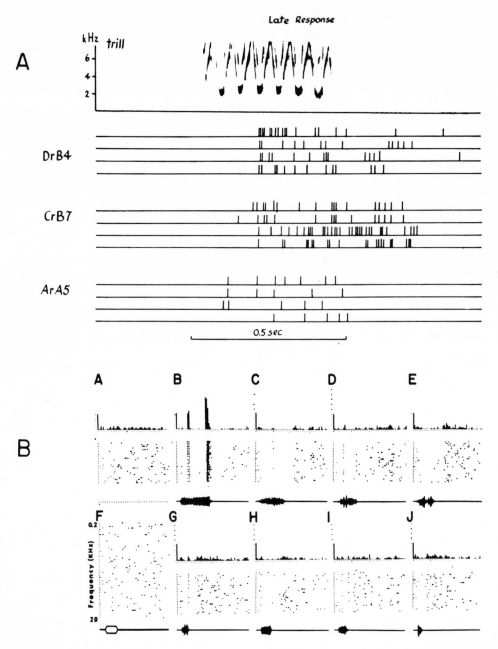

FIGURE 9 Responses of neurons in auditory cortex of squirrel monkey to the species-specific vocalizations. A: 3 neurons responding only to "trill" calls. *Above*: spectrogram of call. *Below*: discharge patterns of each neuron to 4 repetitions of the recorded vocalizations. (From Winter, 1972.) B: Neuron responding selectively to one out of 8 types of vocalization and not to tones. *Lower trace* in each case: envelope of stimulus. *Middle plot*: "dot" display of time of neuronal spike discharge during each of the 25 presentations of the same stimulus making up the average time histogram of the activity over a 2.4 sec sweep, shown in the upper plot. Plot A: spontaneous activity. Plot B: strong excitation by isolation peep call. Plots C to E, Plots G to J: no excitation by err, twitter, err-chuck, rough cackle, shriek, peep and vit calls, respectively. Plot F: "dot" display of results of tone stimulation frequencies between 0.2 and 20 kHz (no discernable response). (From Wollberg and Newman, 1972; copyright 1972 by the American Association for the Advancement of Science.)

temporal patterning, and spectral/temporal complexity and location of auditory stimuli, whereas the ability to discriminate differences of frequency and intensity *per se* are affected little or not at all (reviewed by Neff and Gold-berg, 1960; Neff, 1961). In the cat, bilateral ablation of the primary auditory cortex (AI) alone produces severe deficits in the performance of two-tone pattern discriminations (i.e., high-low-high versus low-high-low) and small but significant degradation of performance in spatial localization tasks (Neff, 1968). Enlargement of the area of ablation to include the primary and secondary auditory areas on both sides (i.e., AI, AII, Ep; for locations, see Woolsey, 1960), eliminates completely tone pattern discrimination and produces severe impairment of the localization of sounds in space. The inclusion of the insulotemporal area (IT) and suprasylvian gyrus in the bilateral ablations rendered the latter deficit complete. Bilateral loss of all auditory areas (AI, AII, Ep, IT, and the auditory area in the second somatic cortex, SII) produces complete loss of the ability to discriminate between tones of differing durations (Sharlock et al., 1965), as well as to localize sounds in space and to detect differences in the temporal patterning of tones. In addition, Kelly and Whitfield (1971) found that lesions of this extent produced a substantial deficit in the ability of cats to relearn to discriminate between the direction of frequency modulation of tones, i.e., the frequency of which were swept in an upward versus a downward direction. Cranford et al. (1971) have recently demonstrated a defect produced by *unilateral* ablation of auditory cortex, namely, the inability of cats to lateralize dichotically presented pulse pairs in a contralateral-ipsilateral (relative to the lesion) sequence to the contralateral ear. On the other hand, bilateral ablation of the primary and secondary auditory areas does not affect the ability of cats to make fine discriminations of differences in tone frequency and intensity. Meyer and Woolsey (1952) found that extending the area of ablation to SII eliminated their previously obtained differential response for frequency, but this failure turned out to be related to the training paradigms used (Thompson, 1960). Thus, later workers are agreed that normal discrimination limina for tone frequency and intensity can be obtained in cats in spite of the bilateral absence of AI, AII, Ep, IT, and SII (see Neff and Goldberg, 1960; Diamond, 1967; Oesterreich et al., 1971). Furthermore, measurements of pitch generalization in the cat before and after bilateral ablation of auditory cortex revealed no significant differences between preoperative and postoperative performance (Diamond, 1967).

Many of these results have been duplicated in the monkey (see Neff and Goldberg, 1960). In addition, in the Rhesus monkey, Dewson et al. (1969) were able to demonstrate that bilateral ablations of the auditory cortex eliminated the ability to relearn and retain discrimination between two vowel sounds, /i/ versus /u/, equated for intensity, whereas the animals could still discriminate tones from broad-band noise. Lesions to the temporal lobes in man also produce sensory deficits analogous to those described above. These produce impairment of localization of sounds in the contralateral acoustic field (Sanchez-Longo and Forster, 1958). Furthermore, lesions of the left temporal lobe in right-handed individuals impair the perception of speech, and lesions of the right lobe can produce loss of the discrimination of differences in timbre, and tonal sequence and pattern. Discrimination limina for frequency and intensity on the other hand are unaffected (summarized in Kimura, 1961).

There is thus a sufficient body of data from the study of single neuron behavior and of the results of cortical lesions to justify the continuation of the search for putative feature abstracting elements in the auditory system, and the mechanisms giving rise to them. We may not be able to substantiate the optimism of some who would see feature-sensitive elements providing the building blocks of such auditory processes as the recognition of music (Deutsch, 1969), but we may be able to uncover something of the "prewired" organization of the auditory system.

Finally, it should be emphasized that, in contrast to the single neuron studies of the visual system, investigations of neuronal properties in the auditory cortex have been almost entirely restricted to the primary projection area. What evidence has already emerged from the relatively restricted number of systematic studies at this level should encourage auditory physiologists to look with more sophisticated stimuli for elements and neuronal assemblies capable of feature extraction, particularly in the areas of auditory cortex as yet unexplored.

ACKNOWLEDGMENT   I am grateful to Dr. J. P. Wilson for helpful criticism of the manuscript.

REFERENCES

Abeles, M., and M. H. Goldstein, Jr., 1972. Responses of single units in the primary auditory cortex of the cat to tones and to tone pairs. *Brain Res.* 42:337–352.

Adrian, H. O., W. M. Lifshitz, R. J. Tavitas, and F. P. Galli, 1966. Activity of neural units in medial geniculate body of cat and rabbit. *J. Neurophysiol.* 29:1046–1060.

Altman, J. A., 1968. Are there neurones detecting direction of sound source motion? *Exp. Neurol.* 22:13–25.

Altman, J. A., 1971. Neurophysiological mechanisms of sound-source localization. In *Sensory Processes at the Neuronal and Behavioural Levels*, G. V. Gersuni, ed. New York: Academic Press, pp. 221–244.

Bogdanski, D. F., and R. Galambos, 1960. Studies of the auditory system with implanted electrodes. In *Neural Mechanisms of Auditory and Vestibular Systems*, G. L. Rasmussen and W. F. Windle, eds. Springfield, Ill.: Charles C Thomas, pp. 143–148.

Brugge, J. F., N. A. Dubrowsky, L. M. Aitkin, and D. J. Anderson, 1969. Sensitivity of single neurones in auditory cortex of cat to binaural tonal stimulation; effects of varying interaural time and intensity. *J. Neurophysiol.* 32:1005–1024.

Capranica, R. R., and L. S. Frishkopf, 1972. Cited in: *Auditory processing of biologically significant sounds. Neurosciences Res. Prog. Bull.* 10 (1):65.

Cranford, J., R. Ravizza, I. T. Diamond, and I. C. Whit-

FIELD, 1971. Unilateral ablation of the auditory cortex in cat impairs complex sound localization. *Science* 172:286–288.

DE BOER, E., 1969. Reverse correlation II. Initiation of nerve impulses in the inner ear. *Proc. Kon. Nederl. Akad. Wet.* [*Biol. Med.*] 72:129–151.

DEUTSCH, D., 1969. Music recognition. *Psychol. Rev.* 76:300–307.

DEWSON, J. H., III, K. H. PRIBRAM, and J. C. LYNCH, 1969. Effects of ablation of temporal cortex upon speech sound discrimination in the monkey. *Exp. Neurol.* 24:579–591.

DIAMOND, I. T., 1967. The sensory neocortex. In *Contributions to Sensory Physiology*, W. D. Neff, ed. New York: Academic Press, pp. 51–100.

ERULKAR, S. D., 1972. Comparative aspects of spatial localization of sounds. *Physiol. Rev.* 52:237–359.

ERULKAR, S. D., R. A. BUTLER, and G. L. GERSTEIN, 1968. Excitation and inhibition in cochlear nucleus. II. Frequency-modulated tones. *J. Neurophysiol.* 31:537–548.

EVANS, E. F., 1965. Behaviour of neurones in the auditory cortex. Ph.D. thesis. University of Birmingham, England.

EVANS, E. V., 1968. Cortical representation. In *Hearing Mechanisms in Vertebrates*, A. V. S. de Reuck and J. Knight, eds. London: J. & A. Churchill, pp. 272–287.

EVANS, E. F., 1971. Central mechanisms relevant to the neural analysis of simple and complex sounds. In *Pattern Recognition in Biological and Technical Systems*, O.-J. Grusser and R. Klinke, eds. Heidelberg: Springer-Verlag.

EVANS, E. F., 1972. The frequency response and other properties of single fibers in the guinea-pig cochlear nerve. *J. Physiol.* 226:263–287.

EVANS, E. F., and P. G. NELSON, 1966a. Behaviour of neurones in cochlear nucleus under steady and modulated tonal stimulation. *Fed. Proc.* 25:463.

EVANS, E. F., and P. G. NELSON, 1966b. Responses of neurones in cat cochlear nucleus to modulated tonal stimuli. *J. Acoust. Soc. Amer.* 40:1275–1276.

EVANS, E. F., and P. G. NELSON, 1968. An intranuclear pathway to the dorsal division of the cochlear nucleus of the cat. *J. Physiol.* 196:76–78P.

EVANS, E. F., and P. G. NELSON, 1973a. The responses of single neurones in the cochlear nucleus of the cat as a function of their location and the anaesthetic state. *Exp. Brain Res.*, in press.

EVANS, E. F., and P. G. NELSON, 1973b. On the relationship between the dorsal and ventral cochlear nucleus. *Exp. Brain Res.*, in press.

EVANS, E. F., J. ROSENBERG, and J. P. WILSON, 1971. The frequency resolving power of the cochlea. *J. Physiol.* 216:58–59P.

EVANS, E. F., and I. C. WHITFIELD, 1964. Classification of unit responses in the auditory cortex of the unanaesthetized and unrestrained cat. *J. Physiol.* 171:476–493.

EVANS, E. F., and J. P. WILSON, 1971. Frequency sharpening of the cochlea: The effective bandwidth of cochlear nerve fibers. *Proc. 7th Internat. Cong. on Acoustics, Vol. 3.* Budapest: Akademiai Kiado, pp. 453–456.

FEHER, O., and I. C. WHITFIELD, 1966. Auditory cortical units which respond to complex tonal stimuli. *J. Physiol.* 182:39P.

FRISHKOPF, L. S., and R. R. CAPRANICA, 1966. Auditory responses in the medulla of the bullfrog: Comparison with eighth-nerve responses. *J. Acoust. Soc. Amer.* 40:1262.

FRISHKOPF, L. S., R. R. CAPRANICA, and M. H. GOLDSTEIN, JR., 1968. Neural coding in the bullfrog's auditory system: A teleological approach. *Proc. IEEE.* 56:969–980.

FUNKENSTEIN, H., P. WINTER, and P. G. NELSON, 1970. Unit responses to acoustic stimuli in the cortex of awake squirrel monkeys. *Fed. Proc.* 29:394.

GEISLER, C. D., W. S. RHODE, and D. W. HAZELTON, 1969. Responses of inferior colliculus neurones in the cat to binaural acoustic stimuli having wide-band spectra. *J. Neurophysiol.* 32:960–974.

GOLDSTEIN, J. L., 1972. Evidence from aural combination tones and musical notes against classical temporal periodicity theory. In *Hearing Theory*. Eindhoven: IPO, pp. 186–208.

GOLDSTEIN, M. H., JR., J. L. HALL, II, and B. O. BUTTERFIELD, 1968. Single unit activity in primary auditory cortex of unanaesthetized cats. *J. Acoust. Soc. Amer.* 43:444–455.

HALL, J. L., II, 1965. Binaural interaction in the accessory superior olivary nucleus of the cat. *J. Acoust. Soc. Amer.* 37:814–823.

HALL, J. L., II, and M. H. GOLDSTEIN, JR., 1968. Representation of binaural stimuli by single units in primary auditory cortex of unanaesthetized cats. *J. Acoust. Soc. Amer.* 43:456–461.

HELD, R., D. INGLE, G. E. SCHNEIDER, and C. B. TREVARTHEN, 1967–1968. Locating and identifying: Two modes of visual processing. *Psychol. Forsch.* 31:44–62; 299–348.

HIND, J. E., 1972. Physiological correlates of auditory stimulus periodicity. *Audiol.* 11:42–57.

HOUTSMA, A. J. M., and J. L. GOLDSTEIN, 1972. The central origin of the pitch of complex tones: Evidence from musical interval recognition. *J. Acoust. Soc. Amer.* 51:520–529.

HUBEL, D. H., C. O. HENSON, A. RUPERT, and R. GALAMBOS, 1959. "Attention" units in the auditory cortex. *Science* 129:1279–1280.

HUBER, F., 1972. Cited in: *Auditory processing of biologically significant sounds. Neurosciences Res. Prog. Bull.* 10. (1):67.

KATSUKI, Y., N. SUGA, and Y. KANNO, 1962. Neural mechanisms of the peripheral and central auditory systems in monkeys. *J. Acoust. Soc. Amer.* 34:1396–1410.

KATSUKI, Y., T. WATENABE, and N. MARUYAMA, 1959. Activity of and neurones in upper levels of brain of cat. *J. Neurophysiol.* 22:343–359.

KAY, R. H., and D. R. MATTHEWS, 1971. Temporal specificity in human auditory conditioning by frequency-modulated tones. *J. Physiol.* 218:104–106P.

KAY, R. H., and D. R. MATTHEWS, 1972. On the existence in human auditory pathways of channels selectively tuned to the modulation present in frequency-modulated tones. *J. Physiol.* 225:657–678.

KELLY, J. B., and I. C. WHITFIELD, 1971. Effects of auditory cortical lesions on discriminations of rising and falling frequency-modulated tones. *J. Neurophysiol.* 34:802–816.

KIANG, N. Y-S., M. B. SACHS, and W. T. PEAKE, 1967. Shapes of tuning curves for single auditory nerve fibers. *J. Acoust. Soc. Amer.* 42:1341–1342.

KIANG, N. Y-S., T. WATENABE, E. C. THOMAS, and L. F. CLARK, 1965. *Discharge Patterns of Single Fibers in the Cat's Auditory Nerve.* Cambridge, Mass.: The MIT Press.

KIMURA, D., 1961. Some effects of temporal lobe damage on auditory perception. *Canad. J. Psychol.* 25:156–165.

KONISHI, M., 1970. Comparative neurophysiological studies of hearing and vocalizations in songbirds. *Z. vergl. Physiologie.* 66:257–272.

LIBERMAN, A. M., F. INGEMANN, L. LISKER, P. DELATTRE, and F. S. COOPER, 1959. Minimal rules for synthesizing speech. *J. Acoust. Soc. Amer.* 31:1490–1499.

MEYER, D. R., and C. N. WOOLSEY, 1952. Effects of localized cortical destruction upon auditory discriminative conditioning in the cat. *J. Neurophysiol.* 15:149–162.

MILLER, J. M., D. SUTTON, B. PFINGST, A. RYAN, R. BEATON, and G. GOUREVITCH, 1972. Single cell activity in the auditory cortex of rhesus monkeys: Behavioural dependency. *Science* 177:449–451.

MOLLER, A., 1970. Unit responses in the cochlear nucleus of the rat to noise and tones. *Acta Physiol. Scand.* 78:289–298.

MORRELL, F., 1972. Visual system's view of acoustic space. *Nature (London)* 238:44–46.

MOUSHEGIAN, G., A. RUPERT, and M. A. WHITCOMB, 1964. Brain-stem neuronal response patterns to monaural and binaural tones. *J. Neurophysiol.* 27:1174–1191.

MOUSHEGIAN, G., R. D. STILLMAN, and A. L. RUPERT, 1972. Characteristic delays in superior olive and inferior colliculus. In *Physiology of the Auditory System.* M. B. Sachs, ed. Baltimore: National Educational Consultants, pp. 245–254.

NEFF, W. D., 1961. Neural mechanisms of auditory discrimination. In *Sensory Communication*, W. A. Rosenblith, ed. New York: John Wiley & Sons, Chap. 15.

NEFF, W. D., 1968. Behavioural studies of auditory discrimination: Localization of the sound source in space. In *Hearing Mechanisms in Vertebrates*, A. V. S. de Reuck and J. Knight, eds. London: J. & A. Churchill, pp. 207–231.

NEFF, W. D., and J. M. GOLDBERG, 1960. Higher functions of the central nervous system. *Ann. Rev. Physiol.* 22:499–524.

NELSON, P. G., S. D. ERULKAR, and J. S. BRYAN, 1966. Responses of units of the inferior colliculus to time-varying acoustic stimuli. *J. Neurophysiol.* 29:834–860.

OESTERREICH, R. E., N. L. STROMINGER, and W. D. NEFF, 1971. Neural structures mediating differential sound intensity discrimination in the cat. *Brain Res.* 27:251–270.

OONISHI, S., and Y. KATSUKI, 1965. Functional organization and integrative mechanism on the auditory cortex of the cat. *Jap. J. Physiol.* 15:342–365.

PAPEZ, J. W., 1967. *Comparative Neurology*, 1st Ed. 1929. New York: Hafner Publishing Co. Also, The connection of the acoustic nerve. *J. Anat.* 60:465–469.

POLJAK, S., 1926. The connections of the acoustic nerve. *J. Anat.* 60:465–469.

ROEDER, K. D., 1971. Acoustic alerting mechanisms in insects. *Ann. N.Y. Acad. Sci.* 188:63–79.

ROSE, J. E., R. GALAMBOS, and J. R. HUGHES, 1959. Microelectrode studies in the cochlear nuclei of the cat. *Bull. Johns Hopkins Hospital* 104:211–251.

ROSE, J. E., D. D. GREENWOOD, J. M. GOLDBERG, and J. E. HIND, 1963. Some discharge characteristics of single neurones in inferior colliculus of the cat. I. Tonotopic organization, relation of spike counts to tone intensity and firing patterns of single elements. *J. Neurophysiol.* 26:294–320.

ROSE, J. E., N. B. GROSS, C. D. GEISLER, and J. E. HIND, 1966. Some neural mechanisms in the inferior colliculus of the cat which may be relevant to localization of a sound source. *J. Neurophysiol.* 29:288–314.

RUPERT, A. L., and G. MOUSHEGIAN, 1970. Neuronal responses of kangaroo rat ventral cochlear nucleus to low frequency tones. *Expl. Neurol.* 26:84–102.

SANCHEZ-LONGO, L. P., and F. M. FORSTER, 1958. Clinical significance of impairment of sound localization. *Neurology* 8:119–125.

SHARLOCK, D. P., W. D. NEFF, and N. L. STROMINGER, 1965. Discrimination of tone duration after bilateral ablation of cortical auditory area. *J. Neurophysiol.* 28:673–681.

SPINELLI, D. N., A. STARR, and T. W. BARRETT, 1968. Auditory specificity in unit recordings from cat's visual cortex. *Exp. Neurol.* 22:75–84.

SUGA, N., 1964. Recovery cycles and responses to frequency-modulated tone pulses in auditory neurones of echo-locating bats. *J. Physiol.* 175:50–80.

SUGA, N., 1965. Functional properties of auditory neurones in the cortex of echo-locating bats. *J. Physiol.* 181:671–700.

SUGA, N., 1968. Analysis of frequency-modulated and complex sounds by single auditory neurones of bats. *J. Physiol.* 198:51–80.

SUGA, N., 1971. Responses of inferior collicular neurones of bats to tone bursts with different rise times. *J. Physiol.* 217:159–177.

SUGA, N., 1972. Analysis of information bearing elements in complex sounds by auditory neurones of bats. *Audiol.* 11:58–72.

SWARBRICK, L., and I. C. WHITFIELD, 1972. Auditory cortical units selectively responsive to stimulus "shape." *J. Physiol.* 224:68–69P.

THOMPSON, R. F., 1960. Function of auditory cortex of cat in frequency discrimination. *J. Neurophysiol.* 23:321–334.

TSUCHITANI, C., and J. C. BOUDREAU, 1966. Single unit analysis of cat superior olive S segment with tonal stimuli. *J. Neurophysiol.* 29:684–699.

VARDAPETYAN, G. A., 1967. Classification of single unit responses in the auditory cortex of cats. *Neurosci. Trans.* 1:1–11.

VARTANYAN, I. A., 1969. Unit activity in inferior colliculus to amplitude-modulated stimuli. *Neurosci. Trans.* 10:17–26.

VARTANYAN, I. A., 1971. Temporal characteristics of auditory neuron responses in rat to time varying acoustic stimuli. *Proc. 7th Internat. Cong. of Acoustics*, Vol. 3. Budapest: Akademiai Kiado, pp. 401–404.

WATENABE, T., and K. OHGUSHI, 1968. FM sensitive auditory neuron. *Proc. Jap. Acad.* 44:968–973.

WHITFIELD, I. C., and E. F. EVANS, 1965. Responses of auditory cortical neurons to stimuli of changing frequency. *J. Neurophysiol.* 28:655–672.

WICKELGREN, B. G., 1971. Superior colliculus: Some receptive field properties of bimodally responsive cells. *Science* 173:69–72.

WILSON, J. P., and E. F. EVANS, 1971. Grating acuity of the ear: Psychophysical and neurophysiological measures of frequency resolving power. *Proc. 7th Internat. Cong. on Acoustics*, Vol. 3. Budapest: Akademiai Kiado, pp. 397–400.

WINTER, P., 1972. Cited in "Auditory processing of biologically significant sounds." *Neurosciences Res. Prog. Bull.* 10(1):72–74.

WINTER, P., and H. FUNKENSTEIN, 1971. The auditory cortex of the squirrel monkey: Neuronal discharge patterns to auditory stimuli. Proc. 3rd Cong. Primat. Zurich, 1970. Basel: Kruger, Vol. 2, pp. 24–28.

WINTER, P., D. PLOOG, and J. LATTA, 1966. Vocal repertoire of the squirrel monkey (*Saimiri sciureus*), its analysis and significance. *Expl. Brain Res.* 1:359–384.

WOLLBERG, Z., and J. D. NEWMAN, 1972. Auditory cortex of squirrel monkey: Response patterns of single cells to species-specific vocalizations. *Science* 175:212–214.

WOOLSEY, C. N., 1960. Organization of cortical auditory system: A review and a synthesis. In *Neural Mechanisms of the Auditory and Vestibular Systems*, G. L. Rasmussen and W. F. Windle, eds. Springfield, Ill.: Charles C. Thomas. pp. 165–180.

14 Psychoacoustical and Neurophysiological Aspects of Auditory Pattern Recognition

J. P. WILSON

ABSTRACT Pitch perception can be considered as a specific example of spectral pattern recognition. Signals with several frequency components frequently give rise to a sensation of pitch that is anomalous on classical theories of pitch perception. Some experiments giving clues to a possible mechanism are described, together with a model of a neural network for the extraction of pitch information. A system of this kind requires inhibitory interaction in order to reject unstructured signals such as white noise and other patterns with components at inappropriate frequencies.

Pitch perception: Emergence of a pattern recognition theory

As PATTERN recognition models for pitch perception have only recently gained support, a brief review of previous theories is necessary, particularly as it is not clear that these can be rejected completely.

At least three kinds of pitch perception have been claimed. (a) Pitch *height* in mels is based on magnitude estimates and fractionation procedures (Stevens and Volkmann, 1940). (b) *Musical* pitch is based on a logarithmic scale of frequency, so that equal pitch intervals are given by equal ratios of frequencies. (It is considered by some to be a cyclical or helical scale, because frequencies an octave apart are more alike than smaller intervals). (c) *Absolute* pitch is usually considered to be a specific kind of musical pitch perception in which subjects can recognize and name pitch without any standard of reference, though frequently for only one note or on a specific musical instrument (Bachem, 1937). Theories have generally been directed toward the second, i.e., musical pitch perception.

Two kinds of theory have persisted under the general headings of *place* and *volley* theory. Place theories have been based on the principle that the separate frequency components of a signal can be analyzed and "mapped" out along some spatial dimension; for example, along the basilar membrane of the cochlea, so that the pitch perceived depends on the place of maximal excitation along this dimension. In theory such a tonotopic relationship can be preserved at higher levels of the auditory system, and it has been observed by Kiang et al. (1965) in the cochlear nerve and by Rose, Galambos, and Hughes (1959) in the cochlear nucleus of cat.

Against this simple view there is a considerable body of evidence that complex signals with components of high frequency can lead to the perception of low pitches. Schouten in 1940 named this phenomenon the "residue" (see Schouten et al., 1962). This led to the concept of "wave form periodicity detection" where pitch depended on the period between repetitions of certain features of the wave form. For this to be possible, there are two requirements: First, that two or more frequency components should interact at the same place to provide the necessary periodicity, contrary to "place" mechanism requirements that would filter the components into separate channels. Second, that temporal features of this wave form should be preserved up to the level of the auditory system at which analysis takes place. The latter does not necessarily mean that each nerve fiber must respond at the wave form repetition rate, but that over the population the wave form should be preserved. This is the basis of the *volley* theory (Wever, 1949) and requires that nerve impulses, although infrequent, should be at least partially phase locked to the stimulus. There is general agreement, based on both psychophysical and single unit studies, that the limit at which phase locking breaks down must be in the region of 5 kHz. Temporal periodicity mechanisms therefore cannot be responsible for what we hear at higher frequencies. This is also the approximate upper limit of *musical* pitch perception. Unfortunately for the auditory theorist, most of the signals giving a strong pitch sensation can be described either in temporal or spectral terms. This equivalence is of course the basis of Fourier analysis. Much ingenuity has been exercised in devising stimulus situations in which some temporal feature exists

J. P. WILSON Department of Communication, University of Keele, Staffordshire, England

without a spectral correlate (e.g., the pitch of pulsed noise, Miller and Taylor, 1947; Harris, 1963; and dichotic pitch phenomena, Cramer and Huggins, 1958; Fourcin, 1970; and the sweep tone effect in mistuned consonances, Plomp, 1967). These special stimulus conditions, however, lead to very weak sensations of pitch and may be mediated by a different mechanism from that utilized for signals with strong pitch.

Some of the first evidence against periodicity pitch came from the ranks of its proponents: Ritsma (1962) found that a three-component tonal residue had lowest threshold (for side bands) when the components were resolvable, and later Ritsma (1967) that the dominant components for the pitch of a complex signal came not from the region of maximal interaction of components but from a region where they were well resolved. However, the significance of these results was not pointed out until later (Terhardt, 1970; Houtsma and Goldstein, 1972).

In attempting to account for the pitch of nonharmonic residues, de Boer (1956) suggested that for widely spaced components it corresponded to the frequency whose integral multiples resemble the given tones as much as possible (i.e., best fitting harmonic series); he also developed, for closely spaced components, an equivalent temporal model based on fine structure of the waveform. Thurlow proposed a *multicue mediation* theory in 1963, but it did not receive wide support at the time. In this theory he proposed that subjects perceived a low pitch by humming, or imagining that they hummed, a low note whose overtone structure matched the components of the stimulus. Such *active matching* or *analysis by synthesis* has, of course, been invoked in other perceptual tasks. Walliser (1969) proposed an empirical rule that perceived pitch corresponds with the subjective subharmonic of the lowest component of a complex that lies closest to the beat frequency between adjacent components (i.e., closest to the common frequency difference). Terhardt (1970) extended Walliser's observations and incorporated them into a *secondary sensation* model in which a low pitch is mediated by the perception of high-frequency components. This appears to be a passive version of Thurlow's model. Whitfield (1970) pointed out that we normally perceive a complex sound as a unitary experience with a specific pitch. This information is carried by the pattern of active and inactive nerve fibers arising from the frequency spectrum of the stimulus. The absence or distortion of a small part of this pattern should not entirely destroy the normal sensation. Wilson (1970), considering the pitch of broadband *comb-filtered* noise, (i.e., noise with multiple spectral peaks, see Figures 1 and 2), proposed a model based on *matching* the spectral peaks in the stimulus to a *best fitting* harmonic series over the *dominant* region of the spectrum. Although matching might be considered to

imply an active process such as Thurlow suggested, this was not specifically intended. The present account will attempt to highlight the important features of this class of matching model and provide evidence in its support. For simplicity a passive model will be formulated here, as there does not appear to be any evidence favoring an active system.

Pitch perception as pattern recognition: An experimental example

A stimulus consisting of noise plus delayed noise has a power spectrum with a series of evenly spaced peaks and troughs (Figure 1a) with the first peak position and common spacing frequency equal to the reciprocal of the time delay Δt. The pitch elicited by this stimulus corresponds with the frequency of the first peak and, therefore, also with the common difference frequency and the reciprocal of the delay time. If now the spectrum is *inverted* (Figure 1b) by phase inverting either the direct or delayed noise, the common difference frequency and time delay will remain the same but the first peak will be an octave lower. Remarkably, however, the perceived pitch neither remains the same nor falls by an octave, but drops by a small amount. According to Fourcin (1965), this pitch change is in the ratio 7:8, but Wilson (1967) found this ratio to depend upon Δt.

A consideration of the initial frequency analysis of this signal by the auditory system indicates that an intermediate region of the spectrum should be dominant in

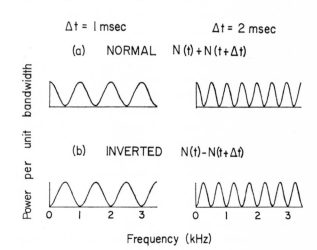

FIGURE 1 Frequency spectra of noise added to delayed noise for delay times (Δt) of 1 and 2 msec. The peaks in the spectral envelopes (a) are harmonically related so that the frequency of the first peak and the common spacing frequency each equal the reciprocal of the delay time ($1/\Delta t = 1$ kHz and 500 Hz). By inverting the phase of one of the noise components the spectral envelope is inverted (b) so that the peaks and valleys of the spectrum are interchanged.

perception. Figure 2 shows spectra similar to those of Figure 1 but plotted on a logarithmic frequency scale to represent better the way in which they are analyzed by the ear. The lower peaks are relatively broad ($\Delta f/f$ large) and cannot be expected to produce a well-defined pitch, whereas the very high peaks, although relatively very sharp, become progressively closer spaced so that eventually the individual peaks cannot be resolved from their neighbors by a system with finite bandwidth filtering as is found in the cochlear nerve (Wilson and Evans, 1971).

If for the moment it is assumed that this dominant region extends from $3/\Delta t$ to $5/\Delta t$ (Figure 2), then the expected pitch ratios can be calculated. On the basis of fitting a harmonic series to the components of the signal in this region, there are two possible series that fit quite closely. One of these has a lower fundamental frequency ($\Delta t' = 9/8 \, \Delta t$) and the other higher ($\Delta t'' = 7/8 \, \Delta t$) giving pitches in the ratios 9:8 and 7:8, respectively, compared with that of the normal spectrum. In order to be able to provide quantitative predictions for pitch, it is necessary to obtain measurements on the extent and location of the region of spectral dominance.

Ritsma (1967) has provided data on dominance for filtered pulse trains. But as all components in Ritsma's stimulus would be sharp and well defined, it is desirable to perform comparable experiments using comb-filtered

noise as the stimulus. Detection threshold was measured rather than the pitch criterion used by Ritsma in view of the possibility that the fourth peak had been found to be dominant because it was a double octave. Subjects were required to determine the detection threshold value of spectral modulation depth by adjustment of the ratio of direct and delayed noise for the whole range of spectral positions and for a variety of spectral peak spacings. The signal was made up from two sources combined through filters. In the first half of the experiment the high-frequency part of the spectrum comprised comb-filtered noise of adjustable peak to valley ratio and the lower part of the spectrum was "filled-in" with noise at the same mean spectral density (see Figure 3, left inset). The

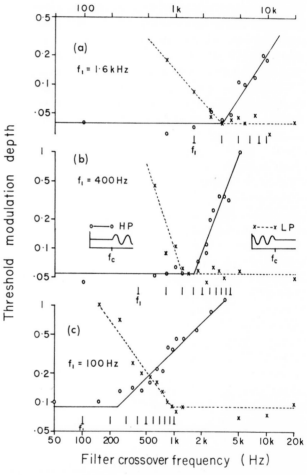

FIGURE 3 Experiments to determine the *dominant* spectral region for three peak spacings (first peak, $f_1 =$ (a) 1.6 kHz, (b) 400 Hz and (c) 100 Hz). The threshold modulation depth (peak to valley ratio of the spectral envelope) measured in the experiment is plotted as a function of the frequency of crossover between a flat spectrum and the comb-filtered noise (see insets that apply to all graphs). The dominant region is that common region where the thresholds obtained under the HP and LP filtered conditions rise (see text). (Reproduced by permission of A. W. Sijthoff.)

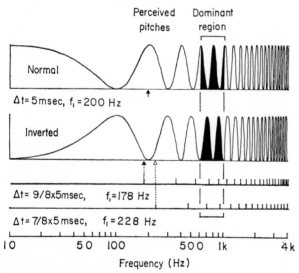

FIGURE 2 Hypothetical scheme to explain the pitch of a *comb-filtered* noise signal. It is assumed to correspond to the fundamental component of a harmonic complex that *fits* the stimulus spectrum over the *dominant* region. These spectra appear different from those of Figure 1, because they are now plotted with a logarithmic frequency abscissa to represent the way they would be *mapped* along the cochlear partition. Below the inverted spectrum are shown two harmonic series that best fit the shaded peaks of the inverted spectrum. Thus the inverted spectrum has a pitch of either 178 Hz or, less frequently, of 228 Hz compared with 200 Hz for the normal spectrum.

threshold peak-to-valley ratio was determined, using a two alternative forced choice (2AFC) technique. With a low value of crossover frequency, f_c, a low threshold was found. Increasing the crossover frequency, however, did not lead to an increased threshold. This means that frequencies between the first and second crossover points were not contributing to the low threshold observed that was determined at a higher frequency region of the signal. Further increments of crossover frequency were made, until eventually a point was found beyond which the threshold increased rapidly. From this it would appear that frequencies above this turnover point were necessary to obtain a low threshold. In the second half of the experiment, the upper and lower parts of the spectrum were interchanged (Figure 3, right inset) and analogous determinations of threshold were made. A turnover point was again found below which the threshold rose. The dominant region is that delimited by the two turnover points. This was repeated for a wide range of peak spacings in addition to those of (a), (b), and (c) in Figure 3.

The mean or optimum dominant frequency is plotted for two subjects as a function of peak spacing in Figure 4. The same data are also expressed as dominant harmonic numbers by reference to the open symbols and right-hand axis. For comparison, Ritsma's mean values are also included. It will be observed that the dominant peak number measured in this way decreases with an increase in the spacing of the spectral peaks. Thus we must expect the pitch difference between the *inverted* and *normal* spectra to become greater as the peak spacing is increased. Measurements of the perceived pitch difference between normal and inverted spectra at two widely separated values of peak spacing, namely at 40 Hz ($\Delta t = 25$ msec) and 1 kHz ($\Delta t = 1$ msec), gave ratios of 1.06 and 1.2, respectively (Wilson, 1967). The corresponding values of dominant peak numbers for these two spacings were 10 and $2\frac{1}{2}$, respectively (Figure 4). This gives predicted pitch ratios of $10:10\frac{1}{2}$ and $2\frac{1}{2}:3$, i.e., 1.05 and 1.2, respectively, in good agreement with measurement.

On the other hand a similar experiment by Fourcin (1965) found the pitch ratio to be approximately 7:8 (1.14) over the frequency range from 110 Hz to 1.2 kHz. This result would be consistent with a *constant* dominant peak number equal to the mean value over this range given by Figure 4. It is possible that Fourcin's subject was listening specifically for this interval. If attention were directed to a particular region of the spectrum, the pitch difference could be expected to correspond to the change

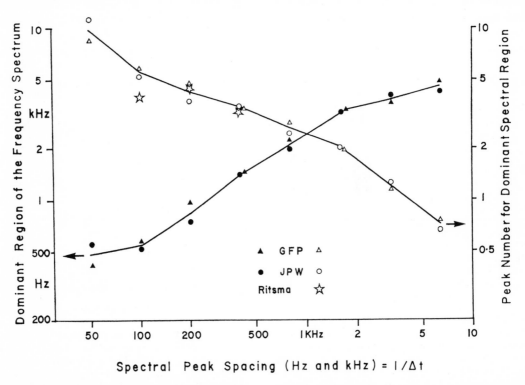

FIGURE 4 Dominant region as a function of peak spacing for two observers. Each point represents a determination such as (a), (b), and (c) of Figure 3. The filled symbols express the dominant regions in frequency terms as spectral position and are referred to the left ordinate. The same data are expressed in terms of the dominant harmonic (peak) number by the open symbols referred to the right ordinate. The mean values obtained by Ritsma (1967) for filtered pulse trains are shown as stars. (Reproduced by permission of A. W. Sijthoff.)

in peak position at that point. This is what Bilsen and Ritsma (1970) found when the range was restricted using filtered signals. They also investigated intermediate shifts in peak position, which gave correspondingly smaller pitch ratios. Although they explained their results in terms of periodicity theory, identical results would be predicted on a pattern recognition model. In the case of high-pass filtering the results would also reduce to Walliser's (1969) rule.

It was seen from Figure 2 that two harmonic series give a good fit to the dominant region of the inverted spectrum. These were obtained by a minimal contraction or expansion of the harmonic series based on 200 Hz and would give rise to pitches corresponding to 178 and 228 Hz, respectively. In fact, both can be observed although the lower one is usually more prominent.

Neural models

In order to account for some of the known properties of pitch perception, a simple neural *pitch unit* can be developed, based on the principle, outlined above, of spectral pattern recognition. Thus if the appropriate harmonically related combination of spectral components is present, a response should occur. At first sight it might appear that inputs to the model could be limited to the dominant region. When the dominant part of the spectrum is removed, however, say by high-pass filtering, pitch can still be perceived. The upper limit may be bounded by what Ritsma (1962) termed the *existence* region of the

tonal residue. The model pitch unit must also be capable of responding to a single pure tone at the fundamental frequency.

Figure 5a shows such a unit in which the frequency spectrum has been mapped into neural space. For simplicity the space dimension has been pictured as linear corresponding to Figure 1 rather than the more realistic logarithmic scale of Figure 2. Such a unit represents one out of a population covering the whole range of possible pitches. The excitatory regions indicated by shading would be determined by the effective bandwidths of the appropriate cochlear nerve fiber inputs (Evans and Wilson, 1971). This simple model would respond to the appropriate signals, but it would also respond to signals that have no pitch such as white noise. To eliminate this it is necessary for the response to be inhibited by the presence of power in the intermediate zones (Figure 5b). Unfortunately, even this system would not be satisfactory, because a single tone at any of the higher harmonies would lead to perception of the fundamental frequency. With the exception of the fundamental input, then, it is necessary to insert a multiplicative process or AND gates so that a response can be obtained only if two adjacent inputs are stimulated simultaneously (Figure 5c). Dominance has not been specifically included in the model shown, but it would be possible to apply either simple weightings, or inhibitory interactions, so that power in the dominant region inhibited responses from surrounding regions.

This model has been derived on the assumption that

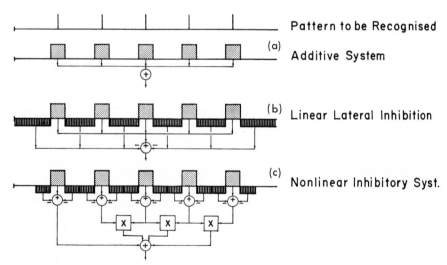

FIGURE 5 Three models for a *pitch unit* for spectral pattern recognition. It is assumed that the spectral pattern to be recognized (a harmonic series in this case) is transformed into neural space according to cochlear analysis and tonotopic organization (upper line). The dotted areas represent excitatory regions corresponding to the effective bandwidths of different regions of

the cochlea and the vertically shaded areas represent inhibition. Addition or subtraction of inputs is indicated by the symbols + and −. Here X represents a multiplicative interaction or the operation of a logical AND gate. For the relative merits of each system see text. Each *pitch unit* represents one out of a population covering the whole range of perceivable pitches.

harmonically related signals are the norm and that non-harmonically related signals are detected by the most closely fitting *pitch unit*. It is, of course, possible to postulate other relationships between the receptors to recognize other spectral patterns of particular biological significance. An obvious example would be for the patterns of formants in speech.

At the moment there is little neurophysiological evidence to support in detail a recognizer of this type (see Evans, in the preceding chapter). There is some psychophysical evidence that the pattern recognizer must be central in location, because Houtsma and Goldstein (1972) found that the pitch sensation from a two-tone complex could still be elicited if the tones were presented separately to the two ears.

Clearly a neural model of this type must become quite complex to accommodate all known properties of pitch perception. It would not have been any easier to develop an active matching model in detail. The general concept of pattern recognition, however, is attractive and allows a given percept to be triggered in a number of different ways. Perception is frequently richer than the stimulus array giving rise to it and depends on learning and prior expectation.

Smoorenburg (1970) found that subjects could be divided into two groups in the way that they perceived a two-component stimulus. If the lower component were reduced in frequency, one group consistently heard the pitch fall whereas the other group heard the pitch rise, presumably corresponding to the consequent increase in fundamental frequency. Individual differences of this kind may also be the basis of the controversy concerning the effect of relative phase of the components on the pitch of a residue. Mathes and Miller (1947) and Ritsma and Engel (1964) reported phase effects in accordance with the requirements of periodicity theory whereas Wightman (1972) reported that he and Patterson had failed to do so in these and other circumstances. Wightman in fact incorporated the latter findings in a pattern recognition model in which the pattern of output of the cochlea undergoes a Fourier analysis. The output of this second stage is then equivalent to an autocorrelation function and a further stage picks the highest peak, which represents the pitch. Such a model, like the present one, is quite insensitive to phase.

In view of the experiments mentioned earlier in which pitch was elicited purely by temporal information (e.g. the pitch of gated noise and dichotic pitch), it would appear desirable to incorporate an additional "box" into the pattern recognition model to allow this. Similar or further boxes may be required for phase sensitivity and the *roughness* detection of Terhardt (1970), and indeed any other attribute that has presumably become associa-ted with pitch through learning. Nevertheless it is only when the ear is denied a pattern of frequency components over the dominant region that it may need to fall back on other such mechanisms.

ACKNOWLEDGMENT   I am grateful to Dr. E. F. Evans for helpful criticism of the manuscript.

REFERENCES

BACHEM, A., 1937. Various types of absolute pitch. *J. Acoust. Soc. Amer.* 9:146–151.

BILSEN, F. A., and R. J. RITSMA, 1968. Repetition pitch mediated by temporal fine structure at dominant spectral regions. *Acustica* 19:114–115.

BILSEN, F. A., and R. J. RITSMA, 1970. Some parameters influencing the perceptibility of pitch. *J. Acoust. Soc. Amer.* 47: 469–475.

CRAMER, E. M., and W. H. HUGGINS, 1958. Creation of pitch through binaural interaction. *J. Acoust. Soc. Amer.* 30:413–417.

DE BOER, E., 1956. On the *residue* in hearing. Ph.D. thesis. University of Amsterdam.

EVANS, E. F., and J. P. WILSON, 1971. Frequency sharpening of the cochlea: the effective bandwidth of cochlear nerve fibres. *Proc. 7th Internat. Cong. Acoustics.* Budapest: Akademiai Kiado, 453–456.

FOURCIN, A. J., 1965. The pitch of noise with periodic spectral peaks. *Rapports 5e Congrès International d'Acoustique*, Liège, Ia, B.62.

FOURCIN, A. J., 1970. Central pitch and auditory lateralisation. In *Frequency Analysis and Periodicity Detection in Hearing.* R. Plomp and G. F. Smoorenburg, eds., Leiden: Sijthoff, 319–328.

HARRIS, G. G., 1963. Periodicity perception by using gated noise. *J. Acoust. Soc. Amer.* 35:1229–1233.

HOUTSMA, A. J. M., and J. L. GOLDSTEIN, 1972. The central origin of the pitch of complex tones: evidence from musical interval recognition. *J. Acoust. Soc. Amer.* 51:520–529.

KIANG, N. Y.-s, T. WATANABE, E. C. THOMAS, and L. F. CLARK, 1965. *Discharge Patterns of Single Fibres in the Cat's Auditory Nerve.* Research Monogram No. 35. Cambridge, Mass.: MIT Press.

MATHES, R. C., and R. L. MILLER, 1947. Phase effects in monaural perception. *J. Acoust. Soc. Amer.* 19:780–797.

MILLER, G. A., and W. G. TAYLOR, 1947. The perception of repeated bursts of noise. *J. Acoust. Soc. Amer.* 20:171–181.

PLOMP, R., 1967. Beats of mistuned consonances. *J. Acoust. Soc. Amer.* 42:462–474.

RITSMA, R. J., 1962. Existence region of the tonal residue. I. *J. Acoust. Soc. Amer.* 34:1224–1229.

RITSMA, R. J., and F. L. ENGEL, 1964. Pitch of frequency-modulated signals. *J. Acoust. Soc. Amer.* 36:1637–1644.

RITSMA, R. J., 1967. Frequencies dominant in the perception of pitch of complex sounds. *J. Acoust. Soc. Amer.* 42:191–199.

ROSE, J. E., R. GALAMBOS, and J. R. HUGHES, 1959. Microelectrode studies of the cochlear nuclei of the cat. *Bull. Johns Hopkins Hospital* 104:211–251.

SCHOUTEN, J. F., R. J. RITSMA, and B. L. CARDOZO, 1962. Pitch of the residue. *J. Acoust. Soc. Amer.* 34:1418–1424.

SMOORENBURG, G. F., 1970. Pitch perception of two-frequency stimuli. *J. Acoust. Soc. Amer.* 48:924–942.

STEVENS, S. S., and J. VOLKMANN, 1940. The relation of pitch to frequency. *Amer. J. Psychol.* 53:329–353.

TERHARDT, E., 1970. Frequency analysis and periodicity detection in the sensations of roughness and periodicity pitch. In *Frequency Analysis and Periodicity Detection in Hearing.* R. Plomp, and G. F. Smoorenburg, eds. Leiden: Sijthoff, 278–290.

THURLOW, W. R., 1963. Perception of low auditory pitch: a multicue, mediation theory. *Psychol. Rev.* 70:461–470.

WALLISER, K., 1969. Uber ein Funktions schema für die Bildung der Periodentonhöhe aus dem Schallreiz. *Kybernetik* 6:65–72.

WEVER, E. G., 1949. *Theory of Hearing.* New York: John Wiley & Sons.

WHITFIELD, I. C., 1970. Central nervous processing in relation to spatio-temporal discrimination of auditory patterns. In *Frequency Analysis and Periodicity Detection in Hearing*, R. Plomp, and G. F. Smoorenburg, eds. Leiden: Sijthoff, 136–152.

WIGHTMAN, F. L., 1972. Pitch as auditory pattern recognition. *Hearing Theory, 1972.* Eindhoven: IPO, 161–171.

WILSON, J. P., 1967. Psychoacoustics of obstacle detection using ambient or self-generated noise. In *Animal Sonar Systems*, R. G. Busnel, ed. Gap, Hautes-Alpes, France: Louis-Jean, pp. 89–114.

WILSON, J. P., 1970. An auditory after-image. In *Frequency Analysis and Periodicity Detection in Hearing*, R. Plomp, and G. F. Smoorenburg, eds. Leiden: Sijthoff, 303–318.

WILSON, J. P., and E. F. EVANS, 1971. Grating acuity of the ear: psychophysical and neurophysiological measures of frequency resolving power. *Proc. 7th Internat. Cong. Acoustics* Budapest: Akademai Kiado, 397–400.

15 Parallel "Population" Neural Coding in Feature Extraction

ROBERT P. ERICKSON

ABSTRACT The development of an understanding of the neural bases of complex neural functions, such as feature detection, is facilitated if a systematic and general understanding of the more primitive processes from which these derive is first established. This chapter is an attempt to examine the extent to which the known "neural" facts of vision, kinesthesis, taste, and so forth may be included under one set of rules, including as guiding principles not only the previously given introspective principles but the known characteristics of neural activity. An initial assumption is that the neural possibilities afforded to one sense by the structure and physiology of its neurons and their connections are also available to the other senses, and thus the encoding parameters available to one are also, to some degree, available to another. This attempt to force the neural processes of all sensory systems into the same small group of mechanisms, by its successes and failures, gives us a view of a general systematic. These principles are then shown to be relevant also to more complex functions, such as feature extraction.

OUR APPROACH to the problem of the neural representation of stimuli in general, including stimulus features, is influenced by at least two very strong and pervasive factors. These influences are radical enough to determine the basic form of our experimental design, as well as the form of our conclusions; thus it would seem reasonable to evaluate these influences from time to time. The first factor concerns our interpretive vocabulary, and the second, our techniques.

Our vocabulary is based on formulations developed by introspective psychologists of the late nineteenth century, mainly Wundt. This formulation was that sensations or perceptions are made up of two kinds of *attributes*, sensory quality and intensity. To these attributes a few others have been added, notable among these being sensory location and duration. The basic requirements for sensory attributes were that variations in each could be accomplished continuously without variations in another (i.e., that they were independent) and that each was necessary for a perception, (i.e., if any one was reduced to zero the sensation would not exist).

It appears that modern neurophysiologists have in large degree accepted this formulation in the sense that the neural underpinnings for one attribute of stimulation (location, for example) are expected to be separate and distinct from those of another (quality, for example). However, some stimulus parameters, such as kinesthesis, do not have a clear definition in this system. Also the structure of the system has been loose enough to allow incorporation of other attributes, with their formal relation to the system remaining unclear; stimulus movement is an important example. The acceptance of this system of stimulus attributes seems to be only informal and implicit, but it appears to be our operating system none the less.

I believe that Wundt's effort to provide a framework that could accommodate all sensory systems may continue to be of use at this time. However, I believe that due to Wundt's lack of understanding of neural processes and later tendencies either to leave a good idea alone or to work without a framework, the present concept of attributes may now hinder rather than facilitate work in the neurophysiology of sensation.

We may usefully reevaluate the concept of attributes in the context of a framework for sensory neural functioning in general; the first part of this chapter, which finds its origin in an earlier paper on the neural representation of simple stimuli (Erickson, 1968), will be devoted to such a systematic approach. In the second half, this system is applied to problems of feature extraction.

To reevaluate the concept of attributes, let us cast aside for the moment all the facts known to Wundt and the psychophysicists after him who were concerned primarily with the description and classification of stimuli. We shall turn to the sensory neural data now available and ask if there is not a simple system of rules that might be used to formalize these events. The basic heuristic will be to include together all similar neural activities into classes and, as consistently as possible, to give similar labels and derive similar encoding principles for all members in a class. Stimulus attributes will be defined neurally, and these definitions will account well for stimuli as diverse in complexity as points, features, and objects.

There are two basic assumptions that will be used in this formulation, assumptions that I believe may be made clearly, but beyond which theoretical travel is perilous.

ROBERT P. ERICKSON   Departments of Psychology and Physiology, Duke University, Durham, North Carolina

First, any process of discrimination, including feature extraction, requires that any stimulus may be defined only in terms of a different or changed stimulus: For example, red would not exist without some other color for comparison. Thus the repeated emphasis in this paper will be on changes in or differences between neural states. Second, the minimal neural requirement for representing discriminable stimulus change is that the neural response must in *some* manner be different for the two discriminably different stimuli: Assumptions are often made about the nature of these changes, for example, that they are accomplished by individual *specific* neurons, such as *feature-detector* neurons. However, the nature of these neural changes is unknown, especially those involved in complex processes such as feature extraction, and form the issue of concern here.

In developing this framework, we must keep perspective on a second factor that has guided our research and thinking, the bias introduced by our techniques. The primary guiding methodology in sensory neurophysiology is the microelectrode, and the basic data consist of the responsiveness of individual neurons. Since our data are largely based on the activity of individual neurons, we are encouraged to conclude that the looked-for functions reside in the activity of these structures. That the individual neuron is the appropriate unit of study for some levels of neural function, such as conduction and synaptic transmission, is beyond question. That it is the appropriate unit of analysis for all neural functions, including more complex functions such as feature extraction, is not clear and should be held open to question. To avoid this bias, consideration will be given to the response of populations of neurons as well as those of individual neurons.

Neural definitions of sensory attributes

In this section an attempt will be made to formulate classes of change in neural activity; these classes will be useful in the neural and psychophysical description of stimulus attributes.

With any given stimulus situation, there are many neurons in activity. To describe or classify this activity in a systematic way would seem at the outset a terribly difficult and complex task. However, we may easily note at least two simple and general kinds of changes in the neural activity, following stimulus changes, that would provide information about the basic parameters involved. For one, the general appearance of the activity might remain the same but simply change in amount, growing greater or smaller. The second general type of change would be that the appearance of the activity could change with the total amount remaining the same; the change in

appearance might be either a change occurring within the same population of neurons, or it might involve a partial or total shift to a new population of neurons.

These types of changes certainly do not accommodate all the candidate parameters of relevant change in neural activity, one notable omission being that of the temporal characteristics of the response and the sequence of activity between neurons; these are treated by Werner (later in this part). Nevertheless, this simplified account of neural changes will suffice to show how such a systematization might facilitate our understanding of complex neural processes, such as feature extraction. It will be used to distill all sensory attributes into two general classes, intensity and quality; the latter class will include such diverse categories of sensory function as color vision, temperature, kinesthetic sensitivity, and location, as well as a range of complexities of sensory function including punctate stimuli and stimulus features.

Intensity

The first type of neural change, that of the total amount of evoked activity, is closely related to the attribute of intensity. Intensive attributes are based on stimulus dimensions producing roughly parallel and monotonic changes in the rate of neural response in all involved neurons (as seen below, nonparallel and nonmonotonic changes in the activity of the involved neurons denote qualitative changes).

In most examples, intensive changes relate in a very straightforward way to existing sensory neural data. Several interesting problems arise with the Wundtian view of intensity, a view based on the psychophysical "more or less"-ness of the stimulus.

Temperature and kinesthesis as intensive attributes

In the temperature sense, when stimulus manipulations are accomplished that have usually been understood as increases in intensity, we know that the steady-state neural activity in at least the Aδ fibers is decreasing. An example of this is shown in Figure 1 (derived from Poulos, 1970). The 15 curves show the responses of individual first-order temperature-sensitive neurons in the trigeminal system of the monkey. I refer to such tuning of curves from all sensory systems as *neural response functions* (NRFs) to call attention to the hypothesized basic similarity in their actions and also use the term *just noticeable differences* (JNDs).

As is clear, the more extreme temperatures evoke the least activity, whereas the more central temperatures evoke the most activity. It would appear that to define neural mechanisms, or attributes, in terms of neural activity, we should label the colder and warmer stimuli as *less* intense than the intermediate stimuli. I would like to return to a discussion of this problem in a moment.

A similar problem in this area arises when we consider the kinesthetic sense. Werner (1968) has successfully used kinesthesis as a model of an intensity attribute. In line

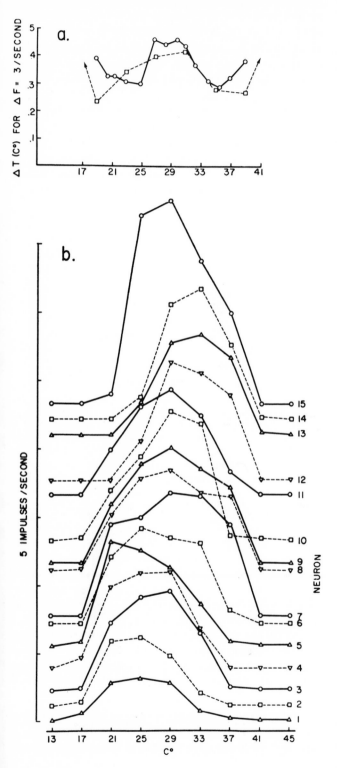

with this view, a number of investigators (Andrew and Dobt, 1953; Boyd and Roberts, 1953; Cohen, 1955; Mountcastle and Powell, 1957; Mountcastle et al., 1963; Burgess and Clark, 1969) have found that as the extremes of extension and flexion are approached, the neural activity increases for some neurons and decreases for others such that some have their maximum rate of response at extension and others at flexion. In Figure 2 are schematically represented the NRFs of individual kinesthetic neurons. For the sake of clarity, only those peaking in activity at full flexion are shown; the mirror-image family of curves, those that peak at extension, has been omitted.

Intuitively, it seems strange to classify kinesthesis as an intensive parameter; common sense would suggest another term such as *position*. However, since these neurons do change their rate of firing monotonically as joint position is varied, the term *intensive* seems a good choice.

Mountcastle et al. (1963) have also shown that the rate of neural response across this parameter follows Steven's power law; this law is very useful in describing intensive functions. However, considering both those neurons that give their greatest response at flexion and extension, it is not clear that the *total* neural input increases as either of these extremes is approached. Therefore, to classify kinesthesis as an intensive continuum at least raises some questions; I would like to discuss this further when I return to considerations of the temperature sense.

Quality

The second major case of neural changes that we observe are those in which the general "appearance" of the neural activity changes; these will be referred to here as changes in the stimulus attributes of quality. The appearance changes because the neurons are tuned in a nonmonotonic and nonparallel manner along their parameters.

FIGURE 1 (a) Solid line: amount of temperature change necessary to produce a JND. After 8 min adaptation, two subjects' difference limens between the hands were obtained by the method of constant stimuli. Peltier refrigerators were used as temperature stimuli for each hand. (Erickson, unpublished.) Dashed line (derived from lower part of figure): amount of temperature change necessary to produce a constant change (here, three impulses/second; arbitrary) in the population of neural response functions given below. (b) Responses to steady temperatures of 15 first-order temperature-sensitive neurons from the face of the monkey (redrawn from Poulos, 1970); extrapolated to 13°C and 45°C. The response function for each neuron is displaced along the ordinate for clarity of illustration; the end points for each curve represent zero impulses/second.

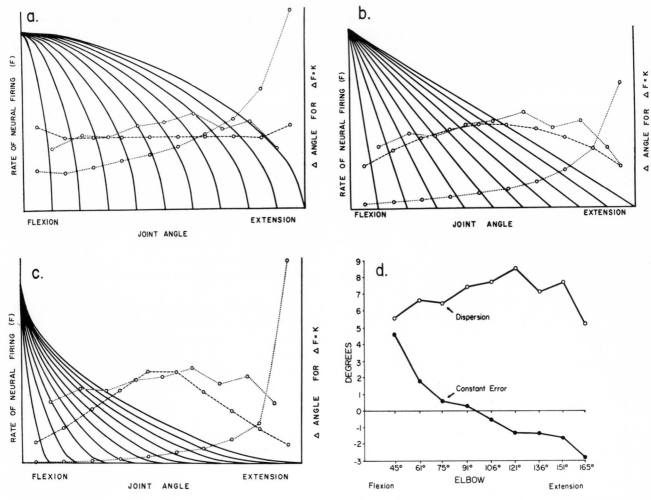

FIGURE 2 (a, b, c) Neural coding of joint positions. *Solid lines:* three probable forms of neural response function (NRFs) of individual kinesthetic neurons (see text for reference). Only those peaking in activity at flexion shown: for clarity, *extensor* neurons not shown. *Dotted line with open circles:* JND curves based on equal changes in the NRFs as in Figures 1 and 5. Curve peaking at *extension* derived from *flexion* NRFs shown. *Dashed line with open circles:* curves derived from the population of both *extensor* and *flexor* NRFs. In b and c, better discrimination is predicted towards the end of the continuum. *Dotted line with* *closed circles:* Identical in a, b, c; also appears in d. Experimentally determined reliability of localization of elbow joint in humans. Note correspondence with derived curves based on both flexors and extensors. (Erickson, unpublished.) (d) *Accuracy of positioning of human elbow.* The six subjects were asked to duplicate the position of one arm with the other arm. The *average* position taken is given as the *constant error* from the correct position. The reliability (standard deviation) is given as the *dispersion;* this curve also appears in a, b, c. Reliability is greatest towards the ends of the dimension. (Erickson, unpublished.)

Erickson has described two general overlapping classes of stimulus quality coding, topographic and nontopographic (1968). In the nontopograpic modalities, broad sensitivity of individual neurons along the relevant dimension (as color coding in visual neurons) is necessary to accomplish the representation of the complete dimensions with a few neurons. In the topographic modalities (as "locations" in vision or in somesthesis) the large quantities of available neurons permit narrow tuning of each. Their inclusion together here as stimulus qualities derives from the similarities in their encoding processes detailed below.

Quality coding: nontopographic

HUE AS A NONTOPOGRAPHIC QUALITY   A classic example of nontopographic quality coding would be that occasioned by changes in the wavelength of the stimulating light. If the position and intensity of the visual stimulus are held constant with only the wavelength varying, then it is approximately true that the same population of neurons will respond, but the general appearance or profile of the activity across these neurons will be modified. That this *across-fiber pattern* (Erickson, 1968) will adequately encode the wavelength of the stimulus follows the logic of Helmholtz (and Hering, for that matter).

In neural terms, this general plan is that hue is represented by certain *relative amounts of activity within a small population* of broadly tuned color-coded neurons. This is illustrated in Figure 3a in which the three NRFs characterize the activity elicited in three types of color-coded neurons; whether these curves are of this particular form or some other broadly tuned form (e.g., opponent process cells) is not of importance here. In Figure 3b is shown the fact that the wavelength of the stimulus is confounded within any one neural element (and may be confused with intensity changes). In Figure 3c it is shown that the wavelength is clearly encoded when the relative activity among the neurons of the population, the across-fiber pattern, is considered; a unique population response obtains for each wavelength-intensity combination. The

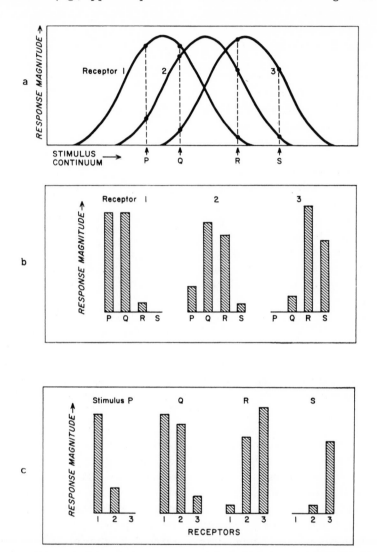

FIGURE 3 Afferent fiber types and patterns of neural activity. (a) Afferent fiber types (or receptor types). NRF curves 1, 2, and 3 represent the responsiveness of three hypothetical afferent fiber types (or receptor types) along a hypothetical stimulus dimension. *P, Q, R,* and *S* represent four stimuli along this stimulus dimension. The responsiveness of a fiber type to one of these stimuli is indicated by the intersection of the response curve and the ordinate erected as the stimulus. (b) Responsiveness of the three fiber (or receptor) types to the four stimuli in (a). In each of the bar graphs is shown the responsiveness of one of the three types to each stimulus in (a). One neuron cannot adequately represent a stimulus, that is, it cannot differentiate between stimuli, because equivalent responses can be given to different stimuli (response of receptor 1 to stimuli *P* and *Q*), and the variations in response magnitude could also be affected by variations in stimulus intensity. (c) Across-fiber patterns. In these bar graphs are shown the patterns of activity across the three fiber types produced by the four stimuli in (a). Each stimulus produces a characteristic pattern across the three fiber types. There would be as many across-fiber patterns as stimuli. With changes in stimulus intensity, the height of the pattern changes but not its form. The quality of stimulus is given in the form of this pattern across a population of neurons. (From Erickson, 1963.)

differences between the four across-fiber pattern responses shown in Figure 3c indicate what is meant in the present context by the encoding of qualitative changes within the same population of neurons.

This view shares similarities with Rock's (1970) speculations about the act of perception in which the meaning of the activity of any neuron is clear only after a "taking account" of the activity of other neurons. This is another way of stating Helmholtz's view that in the sensation of hue, the meaning of the activity of the *red* neurons is only clear after an evaluation (or "taking account") of the activity of the *green* and *blue* neurons. Many others have expressed similar views (for example, Adrian et al., 1931; Hahn, 1971; Hartline, 1940; Mountcastle, 1966, 1968; Mesarovic and Macko, 1969; Poggio et al., 1969; Spinelli et al., 1970; Tower, 1940, 1942; Vastola, 1968; Wright, 1947; Bishop, 1970; O'Connell and Mozell, 1969).

Following Wundt's definition closely, stimulus wavelength changes with the accompanying changes in perceived hue have classically been considered to be an example of the stimulus attribute of quality. He specified that stimulus quality changes should be capable of occurring without changes in any other attributes, such as intensity or duration, and that they should be capable of being accomplished without any discontinuities. Thus, in color, we may move from red through orange and green to blue smoothly and without interruption, and without changes in the other attributes.

TEMPERATURE AND KINESTHESIS AS NONTOPOGRAPHIC QUALITIES   Now I would like to return to a consideration of the problem of temperature and kinesthesis earlier left unresolved. I would first like to point out the general similarities between the NRFs along the temperature dimension (Figure 1) and those of the color-coded neurons along the wavelength dimension (Figure 3). In both cases, each NRF is broadly tuned across the dimension, and its peak activity occurs toward the center of its range. Perhaps, then, the neural coding processes in these systems share some similarities. If true, then the rubric most useful for psychophysical and neural analysis for the temperature sense might be the same as the rubric used for color coding, i.e., sensory quality.

The analysis suggested here for color coding, following the leads of Helmholtz and Hering, will thus be applied to temperature coding; the difference between two temperatures will be presented as neurally and psychophysically analogous to the differences between two colors. What is to be derived is the neural situation obtaining for different temperatures, analogous to the neural situations for differing color codes in Figure 3. This analysis can be obtained from the NRFs of Figure 1 as is

shown in Figure 4 for several different temperatures. In this figure is shown the amount of activity in each of the 15 neurons of Figure 1 at a given temperature; each temperature produces a distinctive pattern of neural activity across this population of neurons.

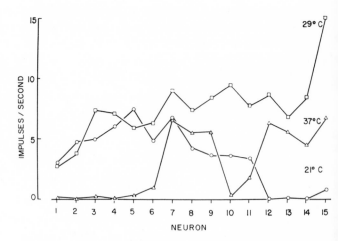

FIGURE 4   Neural representation of temperature. The data points and neuron numbers are from Figure 1. Whereas in Figure 1, the data are presented by neurons, here they are presented by temperatures. This population response, or *across-fiber pattern*, should signal the quality of the stimuli, i.e., the temperature.

That the stimulus changes in hue and temperature are similarly given by the change in the across-fiber pattern, suggesting a communality of the encoding process, may be shown in relation to Figures 1 and 5. Hypothesizing that a JND along these dimensions requires a certain constant amount of change in the population response (Erickson, 1968), the size of the step taken along these dimensions to give a constant change in response is plotted below the curve for the receptor processes in Figure 5; the same derivation may be obtained from data published on opponent-process color-coded neurons. The familiar *w*-shaped function depends on the fact that the size of the step for the constant change in neural activity need not be as large where the slopes of the receptor function are great. For temperature, the same type of derivation is shown in Figure 1a where the two minima of the *w*-shaped function correspond with the more steeply sloping parts of the neural functions. Included also with this is a JND curve obtained psychophysically from the skin of the hand of human subjects. The correspondence between the derived and experimentally determined functions suggests that a similar across-fiber pattern analysis of the quality code is occurring in both cases.

To return to kinesthesis, as illustrated in Figure 2, these NRFs seem to be something like a reversal of the temperature or color-coded NRFs; that is, they show the

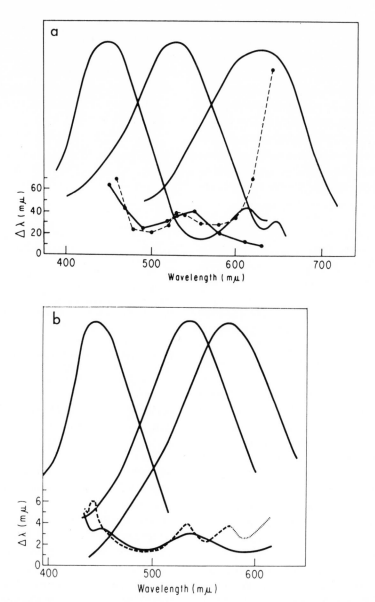

FIGURE 5 Comparison of color JND curves derived from changes in receptor across-fiber patterns with behaviorally determined JND curves. (a) Goldfish. Trichromatic receptor NRFs, from Marks (1965). Dashed curve: derived from receptor NRFs, giving changes in wavelength ($\Delta\lambda$) necessary to produce a constant total change across all three receptor types. Solid curve: behaviorally determined JNDs for goldfish (Yarczower and Bitterman, 1965). Note correspondence between derived and behaviorally determined JND curves (except at long wavelengths). (b) Humans; as upper portion of figure. Receptor NRFs from Marks et al. (1964). Behavioral JND curve from Wright (1947). Note correspondence between general form of JND curves (except at long wavelengths).

same general tuning characteristics except that their peaks are at the extremes of the continuum rather than at the center. There are striking similarities in the types of neural changes occurring with joint movement and with changes in color or temperature stimuli. As the stimuli are varied, the *total* amount of neural activity across all involved neurons varies slightly, but not monotonically as would be expected with intensive changes; the most striking change is in the relative amounts of activity within the population of responding neurons. In this particular case the major changes would be in the pattern of activity between the two general classes of neurons, the extensors and the flexors; these would be analogous in action to two classes of color-coded neurons, or two classes of temperature neurons. This would classify kinesthesis with color and temperature as a qualitative sense.

ROBERT P. ERICKSON   161

We would have our choice here either of considering the neural activity from the joint as two intensive parameters (flexion and extension, and perhaps rotation), or as one qualitative parameter. The qualitative parameter is perhaps more appropriate, because the analysis appears to be that of *comparison* of the activity among all participating neurons, rather than an analysis of one population of these neurons *or* the other. In Figure 2 is shown an analysis of the JND function that would occur considering flexors or extensors alone, and an analysis of the population response analogous to those done of the population response in Figures 1 and 5 for temperature and color. In each part of Figure 2 are shown two derived JND functions, one depending simply on one population of neurons, and one that would derive considering both extensor and flexor neurons simultaneously. Considering only one group of neurons, in each of the three types of curves given (Figure 2a, b, c) the discrimination would become extremely poor at one end of this dimension. Considering both families of neurons, it can be seen that although the JND function would depend on the exact form of the kinesthetic NRFs, it would be much flatter across the continuum than if it were based on only one family of these NRFs. The kinesthesis JNDs that we have derived psychophysically (human elbow) are also shown in Figure 2a–d. The similarity of these "flat" JND functions to those derived from a *population* response of flexors and extensors simultaneously suggests that both families of these neurons are used in the analysis. The most likely form of the NRFs is also suggested, i.e., that shown in Figure 2b or c where discrimination would be better at the extremes of the continuum rather than Figure 2a, where discrimination would be poorer at the extremes.

This suggests that the analysis occurs in a manner similar to that for color and temperature, and that for a simple systematic approach to neural function, kinesthesis should be grouped with them as a qualitative modality.

TASTE AS NONTOPOGRAPHIC QUALITY   A number of facts point to differences between tastes as representing sensory quality in a nontopographic manner (see Erickson, 1968, for review). In mammals in general, each stimulus activates nearly all receptors with which it comes in contact, and each neuron is sensitive to nearly all taste stimuli. Small populations of neurons, those serving one taste papilla for example, are capable of carrying the message for a variety of tastes (Harper, Jay, and Erickson, 1966); this would be expected with each neuron being broadly tuned, and the aggregate of neurons functioning in an across-fiber pattern manner (Figure 6) as in the color system. Also, although diffuse regional differences in sensitivities to various tastes occur across the tongue, and

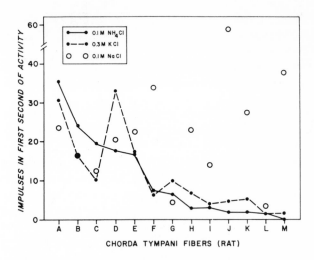

FIGURE 6   Coding of taste quality in a population of neurons. These records from 13 chorda tympani neurons in the pentobarbital anesthetized rat are typical of several hundred obtained. Each neuron responds to all three stimuli, and thus responses in any individual neuron are equivocal with respect to taste quality. The across-fiber pattern of response to each stimulus (at various intensities) uniquely expresses that stimulus. (From Erickson, 1963; see Erickson 1968, Ganchrow and Erickson 1970, and Doetsch and Erickson 1970, for reviews.)

perhaps across areas of neural tissue, the point of stimulation is not a primary cue to the identification of taste quality as would be expected in a topographic system.

SUMMARY   It appears that in order to treat systematically the neural activity resulting from stimulus changes, certain classes of changes may be conveniently grouped together on the basis of their similarities. These include color, temperature, taste, and kinesthetic stimulus changes; other possible sensory mechanisms in these categories not discussed here may include auditory pitch (see below), olfaction (O'Connell and Mozell, 1969), and vestibular sensitivity. The main requirements for this type of stimulus coding are that they may occur within the same set of neurons, that they may occur continuously along their dimension, that they need not be accompanied by intensive changes, and that the main change encoding the stimulus occurs in the pattern of activity evoked across the population of responding neurons (*across-fiber pattern*). The term used here for such change is sensory *quality*. Since these changes do not necessarily require changes in the sets of neurons involved, they are considered nontopographic quality changes.

Quality coding: topographic

The second major class of changes of neural activity involving a change in the "appearance" of the neural activity is that in which there is a partial or total change in the population of neurons involved. The proportion of neurons changed in the two neural situations may vary continuously from no change (which would be the non-topographic class of events just discussed), through slight amounts of change in the population, to a complete change to another set of neurons. *That these types of changes are not entirely disjoint will be emphasized here.* Due to the similarity in the encoding processes, both of these types of neural change will be included under the general classification of "qualitative" changes. With the population of neurons involved changing, we may note a movement of the locus of activity across the neural sheet, such as occurs with movement of the visual stimulus across a visual field or movement of a mechanical stimulus across the skin; these stimulus changes may thus be termed topographic. Since the previously discussed group of neural changes did not involve such a movement across the neural sheet (the change may be accomplished within the same set of neurons), they were termed nontopographic.

TOPOGRAPHIC QUALITY IN AUDITION Auditory coding frequency was previously suggested as a *topographic* qualitative system (Erickson, 1968). At the cortical level, frequency coding may be more appropriately placed in the *nontopographic* group. Several considerations prompt this suggestion. The NRFs for frequency in audition seem to be very broad, at least hazy, at the cortical level. Also, the tonotopic organization of the neural tissue, at the cortical level, appears to be very rough. Perhaps this tissue is given in the topographic way to auditory localization, the rough tonotopic organization seen there being a reflection of an appropriate high-frequency sensitivity for the stimuli in the area of the neuron's sensitivity—on the close side. Narrow tuning for location rather than frequency could be expected of these neurons.

LOCATION AS TOPOGRAPHIC QUALITY It would undoubtedly be objected that there are not many similarities between neural coding in color vision on the one hand and somesthetic location or visual space on the other and that therefore it is not helpful to include them together under the same general coding classification. For example, it seems more likely that a finely tuned individual neuron could encode topographic location in somesthesis or vision more easily than an individual broadly tuned neuron could encode the nontopographic parameters of color and, thus, that a different mechanism, *specificity*, might be expected for location. However, even in these topographic systems in which the neurons may be narrowly tuned across the stimulus dimensions, the specificity of tuning does not account for the fineness of discrimina-

tion any better than it does for hue; discriminations can be easily made over much smaller ranges than the width of the NRFs. Perhaps in both cases discriminability depends upon certain constant amounts of change in the across-fiber patterns encoding the stimuli, independent of the width of the NRF (discussed in Erickson, 1968).

An example of what is meant by coding of this nature in somesthesis is given in Figure 7. These records were obtained from first-order neurons from the forepaw of the rat. Here it is seen that stimuli at two different locations may be encoded by the relative amounts of activity of the population of neurons responding. Stimulus location and intensity are confounded in the activity of any given neuron but are unequivocally given in the population response. Many previous investigators, for over three decades (for example, Adrian et al., 1931; Tower, 1940, 1942), have advocated this kind of analysis in somesthesis. In this, the coding is identical to that in the nontopographic systems.

It is relevant to point out here that Hartline et al. (1961), in an analysis similar to that given for somesthesis above, were able to disclose aspects of neural activity related to spatial edge effects through inferences about relative amounts of activity across a population of neurons.

SUMMARY The main point to be made here is that the coding process in the topographic systems does not appear to be entirely distinct and different from that in the nontopographic systems. In our search for a general simple vocabulary to account for observable neural changes that accompany stimulus changes, we have the choice either of specifying these two types of coding as different, i.e., quality and location, or of taking note of the similarities of the coding process as seen from the point of view of the nervous system, and including them together as two subtypes of the same coding process, that of stimulus quality.

It is interesting to note here that *stimulus location* follows closely the definition set forth by Wundt for stimulus quality; that is, changes may be made along this stimulus dimension in a continuous fashion and independent of other stimulus attributes. It may have been our concern with the physical description of the stimulus, rather than a clear difference in neural process, which has led us to deal with location and quality as involving separate sensory mechanisms.

Coding for other neural functions

Before bringing this rather simple formulation to bear on the problem of feature extraction, I would like to point out one other result of this systematization of neural

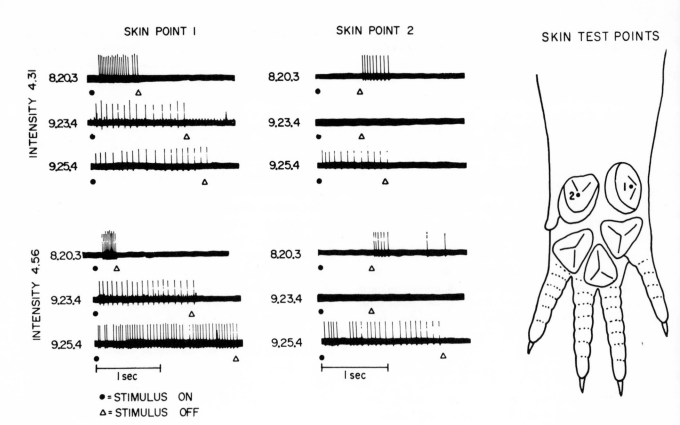

SKIN POINT I   SKIN POINT 2   SKIN TEST POINTS

INTENSITY 4.31

8.20.3

9.23.4

9.25.4

INTENSITY 4.56

8.20.3

9.23.4

9.25.4

1 sec   1 sec

●= STIMULUS ON
△= STIMULUS OFF

FIGURE 7 Parallel neural coding of stimulus location and intensity in somesthesis. Responses of three (representative of recordings from 50) individual neurons in the median nerve of the phenobarbital anesthetized rat to graded stimulation by von Frey hairs (Semmes and Weinstein, et al., 1960) at two skin locations. The rate of response of any individual neuron may be similarly influenced by changes in location, intensity, and in some cases (neuron 8.20.3) in timing—stimulus *on* vs. *off*. However, considering all three neurons together, there is an unequivocal representation of position, intensity, and timing. (Cassel and Erickson, unpublished.)

activity. The neural changes in a sheet of neural tissue involved in motor response (see Figure 8, part 3) and those in a sensory sheet (see Figure 8, part 1) are thus seen to involve many similarities. To classify movements neurally, many parallel neurons would be in activity for each movement. That is, no movement, at any neural level, is ever represented by activity in one neuron or one group of neurons; at the very least, a complex pattern of activity in flexors and extensors is involved. As the organism changes from one movement to another, the general across-fiber pattern of activity of many efferents would be seen to shift in amplitude and shape.

I make these suggestions for several reasons; first, on the intuitive level it would be rather surprising if the nervous system evolved different principles of encoding mechanisms for sensory and motor functions—it would be uneconomical in light of the similarities of the machinery used (neurons and their interconnections). Other functions such as memory storage or other biasing mechanisms might also share some of these principles. (See Figure 8, part 2.)

Second, these various functions, i.e., sensation, movement, and memory, face many of the same problems. The basic problem is one of economics; that is, many different events must be expressed with a limited number of neurons. The color system, in which a very few types of color-coded neurons can represent the total wavelength dimension, expresses the solution to this problem admirably. In the motor system, many different movements must be expressed with a limited number of motor neurons. Even in a simple nervous system with *command* neurons, this principle applies (see Davis and Kennedy, 1972). In memory, the problem seems to be particularly staggering. The memories of a lifetime must be represented somehow with a rather limited number of neurons.

Also, in each case, the function is given in a distributed manner to the cooperative responsibility of many neurons, and thus each function has the neural safety and weight of being expressed by a large portion of the brain. It is to be noted that although this distributed manner of coding gives each function the mass action and equipotentiality of a hologram, the similarities do not necessarily include

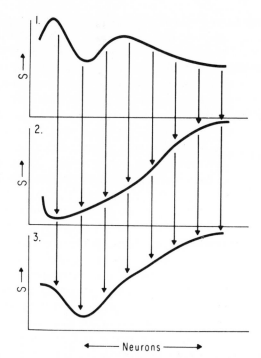

FIGURE 8 General conception of the form and interrelationships of the representations of neural events at several levels. Ordinates give level of activity (e.g., graded potentials, biochemical state) of the neurons represented along abscissa. Coding at all levels takes the same general parallel "population" form, and influences from one level to the next are also parallel. The intermediate level 2 represents mechanisms such as memory storage and motivational states, modifying the response 3 to the input level 1. The level 3 is any efferent or resultant function, such as perception or movement. The presence of convergence, divergence, feedback, etc. does not qualitatively alter the general form of the coding process and is not illustrated.

the mechanisms producing these effects (see Gabor, 1972).

Finally, if the same general principles are utilized by these several interlocking processes, then there need be no change in the general *form* of the message from one level to another. For example, the nervous system need not change the form of its information for the purpose of intermediary *gnostic* or *pontifical* neurons.

These considerations are not entirely novel; some have very long histories. They are briefly reiterated here to indicate the generality and feasibility of the proposed mechanism of neural coding.

A final note might be added about the feasibility of studying population responses and the improbability that all functions utilize the same mechanisms. Perkel and Bullock (1969) have suggested that the encoding of sensory events probably depends on a population response but were doubtful about the possibility of the researcher accomplishing such an analysis. It was shown above that such an analysis is only slightly more complex than analysis of the activity of individual neurons and that the latter

may be misleading in the investigation of sensory neural processes.

Concerning the generality of sensory mechanisms, some factors are probably unique to each sensory system. For example, the problem of stereopsis may be unique to vision, the solution of phase-locked volleying and the use of interaural Δt unique to audition, and a descending afferent anatomy unique to olfaction. Still, the nervous system uses much the same neural machinery in all the sense systems and thus probably did not evolve entirely different coding processes for each of them. Their similarities should prove useful, and at least encourage the illumination of one area of sensory neurophysiology by discoveries in other areas.

Application to feature extraction

The general systematic for neural sensory representation presented in the first half of this paper is of use in two problems related to feature extraction. It bears on the question of (1) how stimulus features are represented neurally, and on the issue of (2) the level of feature "specificity" which we may expect from individual neurons participating in feature extraction.

Neural representation of stimulus features

In considering feature extraction, we generally turn to the area of vision. Here, there are certainly more extractable features than in some of the simpler afferent systems. Of the two problem areas of color and form, probably those of color, including adaptation and contrast effects, compose the simplest categories; these are probably encoded simply by the across-fiber pattern of activity within the responding population as suggested by Helmholtz and Hering. The more complex problems of feature extraction probably relate to visual form.

The basic requirements for the encoding of a complex array of visual form is that each form elicits neural responses that differ from others in some respect; this is met by a camera-like nervous system of simple point detectors. Why should there have evolved in the visual system any process of feature extraction more complicated than this?

To approach this problem, let us inspect the utility of some fairly well accepted feature-extractor neurons, the line-sensitive neurons of Hubel and Wiesel. In brief, these central visual neurons respond best to straight lines, and the response of each of these neurons drops off *gradually* as the line is rotated from its best orientation. This situation is schematized in Figure 9 with the representation of the NRFs of three neurons responsive to the orientation of straight lines. Neither the fact that the stimulus was a line nor the orientation of that line is portrayed in the activity of any individual neuron, just as in color vision the wavelength of the stimulus is not unequivally given in the responsiveness of any color-coded visual neuron. Within each neuron, equivalent responses may be obtained at either of two line orientations, and the amount of this response is also influenced by the intensity and the wavelength of the light; thus all stimulus parameters are confounded in any one neuron's response. The neuron will also respond, although to a lesser degree, to points, curved lines, lines of various width and so forth, and complex forms; these latter problems will be returned to after consideration of the coding of the stimulus as a straight line.

The three curves given in Figure 9 were chosen to emphasize the similarities between line-orientation coding and coding in color vision (Figures 3 and 5); the continuity of curves in line coding, rather than being confined to three groups, does not qualitatively influence the argument concerning their similarities, nor does the fact that the breadth of tuning may be somewhat narrower than for color. If this analogy is pursued, the advantages of this type of neural responsiveness are immediately clear: All line orientations and their brightnesses may be encoded by considering the relative amounts of activity across a few neurons. Thus, coding for line orientation could to great advantage follow the same principle as seen for color vision, temperature, and other members of the nontopographic quality series.

An example from Figure 9 of how simultaneous encoding of these stimulus features could be supported in a small population of nine neurons is given in Table I. Here unequivocal and simultaneous encoding of stimulus location (given by the topographic identity of the group), intensity,

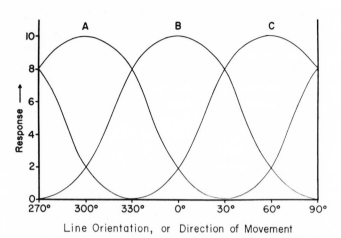

FIGURE 9   Parallel neural coding for all line orientation by three broadly tuned, line sensitive neurons. The mechanism is presumed to be the same as described for the encoding of all visual wavelengths by a few broadly tuned color-coded neurons (see Figure 3). This figure also is used to describe, in a similar manner, the encoding of direction of movement of stimuli in somesthesis and vision. Table 1 is derived from this figure.

TABLE I

Each cell gives the responses of the same nine color-coded neurons with line orientation properties as illustrated in Figure 9. The curves in Figure 9 give the response at the most stimulating wavelength (at intensity). As an example, a red line at 0° orientation (center cell, upper row) stimulates maximally (10) a *red* neuron tuned optimally to 0°. The *green* neuron tuned maximally to 0° would give a lesser response (e.g. 5), and a *blue* neuron still less (e.g. 2.5). (The latter 2 responses not illustrated in Figure 9.) This ratio across R-G-B neurons (10-5-2.5) indicates *red* under all conditions of line orientation and intensity. Changing wavelength to green at the same line orientation (moving from center to right cell) changes pattern across R-G-B neurons to 5-10-5 (G neurons now give maximal response).

Line orientation is given across A-B-C neurons (2-10-2 ratio in upper center cell). This pattern is unchanged in changing wavelength (moving from center to right cell). However, changing orientation but not wavelength (moving from center to left cell) changes only A-B-C pattern, (from 2-10-2 to 8-0-8) leaving color pattern across R-G-B neurons unchanged.

Changes in intensity (moving from upper to lower row of cells) changes level of responding, leaving patterns unchanged.

			Straight-Line Stimulus								
			90° Red			0° Red			0° Green		
	Neurons		R	G	B	R	G	B	R	G	B
Intensity 1	"120°"	A	8	4	2	2	1	0.5	1	2	1
	"0°"	B	0	0	0	10	5	2.5	5	10	5
	"60°"	C	8	4	2	2	1	0.5	1	2	1
Intensity 2	"120°"	A	16	8	4	4	2	1	2	4	2
	"0°"	B	0	0	0	20	10	5	10	20	10
	"60°"	C	16	8	4	4	2	1	2	4	2

hue, and line orientation are condensed into the activities of nine neurons.

To the extent that this example is correct in principle, the breadth of tuning along several stimulus parameters indicates that stimulus features may not be extracted in the activities of individual neurons. Rather, this breadth of tuning makes possible the process of feature extraction by a small population of neurons. Thus, although the stimulus feature of a straight line could be adequately represented by point detectors, it is also adequately represented by a much smaller population of neurons broadly tuned to straight lines.

A major advantage of representing this stimulus feature with a small number of neurons is that it may be represented redundantly over many small populations of neurons and in a distributed manner across neural tissue. Redundancy becomes a major issue in sensory representation. In a camera-like system composed of point detectors, the activity of each neuron is crucial in the representation of the stimulus, and loss of one small point in the sheet of neural "film" would cause distortion of the perceived figure. Due to redundancy of figure representation in the broadly tuned line detector system, poor reliability (in the rate of neural firing), or even neuron loss, becomes much less critical.

The development of multiple neural sensitivities

In an attempt to determine what further or different processes of feature extraction may be expected, let us state the rules that characterize what has happened in the above very simple and concrete example of "feature extraction." At the simpler level we have a stimulus encoding process in which intensity is given by the total amount of activity across the responding population. In addition, one stimulus quality, i.e., location, is encoded topographically with narrowly tuned NRFs and another stimulus quality, i.e., wavelength, is encoded nontopographically with broadly tuned NRFs by the same neurons. It was possible and fruitful to add another sensitivity, that is, the tilt of the straight lines at that point. This process could be characterized simply as the adding of another nontopographic parameter of sensitivity to the NRFs of these neurons.

Without belaboring the encoding of these aspects of stimulus in detail, it may be pointed out that as was the case with line orientation, nontopographic responsiveness along other dimensions such as direction and rate of movement may be added to these neurons. Figure 9, with relabeled axes, may be used to demonstrate coding of direction and rate of movement by the conjoint responses of a few neurons (the abscissa now scales direction of movement; different curve heights would result from different rates of movement). The similarity of neural

coding between stimulus movement and the other sensory qualities would indicate that movement should be classified with them.

In this model, the *simultaneous* activity of a small group of movement-sensitive neurons is used to signal the rate and direction of movement. Considered over time, the postulate that any stimulus aspect could be encoded by *any* differences in neural activity indicates that an adequate code for stimulus movement also resides in the *sequential* activity of point detectors that are not individually sensitive to movement. Werner (later in this part) has also indicated the possible role of movement detectors in the sequential buildup of perceptions from elementary feature detectors.

As long as the additional sensitivities are broadly tuned, then each stimulus (in this example a line of any color, orientation, width, length, curvature, movement, etc.) will evoke a unique response in the *population* of responding neurons, and thus will be adequately encoded. If the neurons become narrowly tuned along any of these dimensions, such as stimulus location, then the size of the population of neurons responding will be limited. If the NRFs along more than one parameter become narrowly tuned, the population response would be severely limited. For example, if neurons were tuned narrowly to both stimulus location and line orientation, or any other pair of dimensions, then the response to any stimulus would necessarily be restricted to a very small number of neurons: The activity in such a system would be close to zero, and we know that this is not the case.

Presumably if narrow tuning along some "new" parameter is introduced at higher CNS levels, as Gross has shown for visual neurons in inferotemporal cortex (Part 3, this volume), then the narrow tuning along other parameters—as *location specificity*—must be abandoned. On the other hand, whenever narrow tuning is abandoned, as Evans has shown for cortical auditory neurons along the frequency dimension (later in this part), then we may expect narrow tuning, possibly with topographic organization, along some other "new" parameter.

To summarize, each neuron may be sensitive along many broadly tuned (nontopographic) dimensions but sensitive to only one narrowly tuned (topographic) dimension.

The development of complex sensitivities

Stimulus features could, in the manner described above, be encoded by any of a large range of complexities of sensitivities. What degree of complexity would be the most effective? Would sensitivity of a neuron to a particular human face be feasible? Probably few neurons would develop such a sensitivity to this stimulus, because this stimulus would not be important enough to a species or occur frequently enough in the experience of an individual to command the sensitivity of a neuron. The occurrence of "face" neurons would be uneconomical, because such neurons would seldom, if ever, be brought into play. They could be considered "stupid" neurons in that their usefulness would be very limited; on the one hand we might equate narrowness of responsiveness with inflexibility (e.g., the fixed and limited usefulness of some narrowly tuned invertebrate neurons), and on the other we might relate breadth of responsiveness with versatility.

At the other extreme of complex sensitivity, a *point-sensitive* neuron would often be in use, responding to any stimulus falling on its receptive field. However, a neuron sensitive to any other common, or frequent, stimulus feature would also be assured an important role in the encoding of visual stimuli. These sensitivities could be of *any* form, but they would have to match common stimuli in the experience of the animal to keep the mass of the neural response high. The mass of neural response to any stimulus must be kept fairly high to make redundancy possible. A great variety of sensitivities would be appropriate for this requirement; however, neurons sensitive to points and approximate line shapes would be, by far, the most numerous, because they would be most heavily activated.

Presumably, these complexities of sensitivities of the visual neurons would develop only because of the complexities common in the stimuli. In kinesthesis and temperature, no further, higher-level processes of feature detection are developed, because there simply are no further useful complexities to be encoded. The feature-extraction process which evolves, then, depends on the useful complexities in the stimulus situation as well as on their frequency of occurrence.

This statement must be modified somewhat, because each species, in the face of a similar world of stimuli, develops different neural sensitivities. Each species evolves its own unique general neural machinery that is maximally useful in its niche. The departure from a point-detecting neural sheet of "film" toward a system selective to important aspects of the stimulus is different for each species. The amount of complexity of sensitivity of the individual neurons would depend both on the number of neurons available and the behavioral requirements of the organism. The frog certainly does not have as much neural tissue to devote to vision as does the cat. If the frog expends these few neurons in the development of complex sensitivities such that heavy inputs occur only for a few specialized stimuli, it does so at the expense of versatility in its output; it has only a few responses related to a correspondingly limited number of classes of stimuli, and this is appropriate for a frog.

Also, since the sensitivities of these neurons may depend to a certain degree upon the experience of the organism

(Spinelli et al., 1972; Blakemore, earlier in this part), the responsiveness developed probably results from whatever neural input has most often been involved (has been "common") in evoking their activity. This would make it probable that each stimulus produces activity in a large population of neurons. The particular sensitivities to aspects of the stimulus may consist of decrements in sensitivity from some innate baseline due to nonoccurrence of a particular feature, or acquisition of sensitivities beyond this baseline due to frequent occurrence of a particular feature, or both. In any case, the final sensitivity suggested here is one that would find the neuron frequently responding to the environment.

Thus, the precise and subtle sensitivities, as influenced by the experience of the organism, are probably impressed upon each neuron's rough innate sensitivities. The thrust of both these processes, evolutionary and experiential, would be to develop neural sensitivities as rich or complex as would be consistent with heavy neural responding to each stimulus of importance to the organism.

From this I would like to suggest that there probably exists a rich array of neural sensitivities, ranging from approximate straight-line sensitivity through increasing levels of complexity, to perhaps a "few" face neurons. The frequency of occurrence of these cells would be greatest for the more simply formed sensitivities, dropping rapidly with greater levels of complexity; face cells would be in a very extreme minority. This progression toward cells of great complexity of sensitivity, however, would not be the process of feature extraction; the feature extraction process would consist of the population response. At no level of specific complexity of response could a neuron by itself be a feature extractor, because the mass of the response and the redundancy would be so critically limited.

Summary

In order to gain perspective on the neural processes of feature extraction, a systematic model for the neural encoding of stimuli was developed; this model was based on the known characteristics of the responsiveness of afferent systems to simple stimuli. The model was incomplete in detail and was used merely to suggest how a systematic approach to problems of feature extraction might be useful.

Within the context of this model, it was concluded that feature extraction is not necessarily as complex a neural process as the complexity of the percept would suggest, i.e., that there may not be an isomorphism of complexity between percepts and neural processes. It may be incorrect to treat as qualitatively distinct such diverse processes as sensory location and classical quality, feature detection, and the perception of objects. All these processes probably depend in a qualitatively similar manner upon the relative amounts of activity of a population of neurons, each member of which would show rather simple stimulus sensitivity, rather than the activity of individual highly complex extractor neurons. It was suggested that in general the sensitivities of the neurons involved in feature extraction would be to rather general and simple stimulus features. The frequency of occurrence of various levels of complexity of sensitivity should be inversely related to the extent of these complexities. Demonstration of the feasibility and usefulness of the analysis of the activity of population of neurons were shown for a variety of sensory systems.

ACKNOWLEDGMENT Supported in part by National Science Foundation research grant GB-33464X.

REFERENCES

ADRIAN, E. D., McK. CATTELL, and H. HOAGLAND, 1931. Sensory discharges in single cutaneous nerve fibers. *J. Physiol.* (*London*) 72:377–391.

ANDREW, B. L., and E. DOBT, 1953. The deployment of sensory nerve endings at the knee of the cat. *Acta Physiol. Scand.* 28:287–296.

BISHOP, P. O., 1970. Beginning of form vision and binocular depth discrimination in cortex. In *The Neurosciences, Second Study Program*, G. C. Quarton, T. Melnechuk and G. Adelman, eds. New York: Rockefeller University Press, pp. 471–485.

BOYD, I. A., and T. D. M. ROBERTS, 1953. Proprioceptive discharges from stretch receptors in the knee-joint of the cat. *J. Physiol.* 122:38–58.

BURGESS, R. P., and F. L. CLARK, 1969. Characteristics of knee-joint receptors in the cat. *J. Physiol.* 203:317–335.

COHEN, L. A., 1955. Activity of knee-joint proprioceptors recorded from posterior articular nerve. *Yale J. Biol. Med.* 28:225.

DAVIS, W. V., and D. KENNEDY, 1972. Command interneurons controlling swimmeret movements in lobster. II. Interaction of effect on motoneurons. *J. Neurophysiol.* 35:13–19.

DOETSCH, G., and R. P. ERICKSON, 1970. Synaptic processing of taste quality information in the nucleus tractus of the rat. *J. Neurophysiol.* 33:490–507.

ERICKSON, R. P., 1963. Sensory neural patterns and gustation. In *Olfaction and Taste*. Y. Zotterman, ed. New York: Pergamon Press, pp. 205–213.

ERICKSON, R. P., 1968. Stimulus coding in topographic and non-topographic afferent modalities: On the significance of the activity of individual sensory neurons. *Psychol. Rev.* 75:447–465.

GABOR, DENNIS, 1972. Holography. *Science* 177(4046):299–313.

GANCHROW, J. R., and R. P. ERICKSON, 1970. Neural correlates of gustatory intensity and quality. *J. Neurophysiol.* 33:768–783.

HAHN, J. F., 1971. Stimulus-response relationships in first-order sensory fibers from cat vibrissae. *J. Physiol.* 213:215–226.

HARPER, H. W., J. R. JAY, and R. P. ERICKSON, 1966. Chemically evoked sensations from single human taste papillae. *Physiol. and Behav.* 1:319–325.

HARTLINE, H. K., 1940. The receptive field of the optic nerve fibers. *Am. J. Physiol.* 130:690–699.

HARTLINE, H. K., F. RATLIFF, and W. H. MILLER, 1961. Inhibitory interaction in the retina and its significance in vision. In *Nervous Inhibition*, E. Florey, ed. New York: Pergamon Press, pp. 241–284.

MARKS, W. B., 1965. Visual pigments of single goldfish cones. *J. Physiol.* 178:14–32.

MARKS, W. B., W. H. DOBELLE, and E. F. MacNICHOL, 1964. Visual pigments of single primate cones. *Science* 143:1181–1183.

MESAROVIC, M. D., and D. MACKO, 1969. Foundations for a scientific theory of hierarchical systems. In *Hierarchical Structures*, L. L. Whyte, A. G. Wilson, and D. Wilson, eds. New York: Elsevier Publishing Company, pp. 29–50.

MOUNTCASTLE, V. B., and T. P. S. POWELL, 1957. Central nervous mechanisms subserving position sense and kinesthesis. *Bull. Johns Hopkins Hosp.* 105:173–200.

MOUNTCASTLE, V. B., G. F. POGGIO, and G. WERNER, 1963. The relation of thalamic cell response to peripheral stimuli varied over an intensity continuum. *J. Neurophysiol.* 26:807.

MOUNTCASTLE, V. B., 1966. The neural replication of sensory events in the somatic afferent system. In *Brain and Conscious Experience*, J. C. Eccles, ed. Berlin: Springer-Verlag, p. 85.

MOUNTCASTLE, V. B., 1968. Physiology of sensory receptors: Introduction to sensory processes. In *Medical Physiology*, vol. II. St. Louis: The C. V. Mosby Co., 12th ed. pp. 1345–1371.

O'CONNELL, R. J., and M. M. MOZELL, 1969. Quantitative stimulation of frog olfactory receptors. *J. Neurophysiol.* 32:51–63.

PERKEL, D. H., and T. H. BULLOCK, 1969. Neural coding. In *Neurosciences Research Symposium Summaries*, vol. 3, F. O. Schmitt, T. Melnechuk, G. C. Quarton, and G. Adelman, eds. Cambridge, Mass.: MIT Press.

POGGIO, G. R., Y. LAMARRE, F. BAKER, and E. R. SANSEVERINO, 1969. Afferent inhibition at input to visual cortex of the cat. *J. Neurophysiol.* 32:892–915.

POULOS, D. A., and R. A. LENDE, 1970. Response of trigeminal ganglion neuron to thermal stimulation of oral-facial regions: 1. Steady-state response. *J. Neurophysiol.* 33:508–517.

ROCK, I., 1970. Perception from the standpoint of psychology. In *Perception and its Disorders*, Res. Publ. Assoc. Res. Nervous and Mental Disease, Vol. 48. Baltimore: Williams & Wilkins.

SEMMES, J., S. WEINSTEIN, L. GHENT, and H. L. TEUBER, 1960. *Somatosensory Changes after Penetrating Brain Wounds in Man.* Cambridge, Mass.: Harvard University Press.

SPINELLI, D. N., H. V. B. HIRSCH, R. W. PHELPS, and J. METZLER, 1972. Visual experiences as a determinant of the response characteristics of cortical receptive fields in cats. *Exp. Brain Res.* 15:289–304.

SPINELLI, D. N., K. H. PRIBRAM, and B. BRIDGEMAN, 1970. Visual receptive field organization of single units of the visual cortex of monkey. *Intern. J. Neurosc.* 1:67–74.

TOWER, S. S., 1940. Unit for sensory reception in cornea. *J. Neurophysiol.* 3:486–500.

TOWER, S. S., 1942. Pain: Definition and properties of the unit for sensory reception. Research Publications. *Assoc. for Research in Nervous and Mental Disease*, 23:16–43.

VASTOLA, E. F., 1968. Localization of visual functions in the mammalian brain: A review. *Brain, Behav., and Evol.* 1:420–471.

WERNER, G., 1968. The study of sensation in physiology: Psychophysical and neurophysiologic correlations. In *Medical Physiology*, vol. II. St. Louis: The C. V. Mosby Co., 12th ed. pp. 1643–1671.

WRIGHT, W. D., 1947. *Researches on Normal and Defective Color Vision*. St. Louis: The C. V. Mosby Co., pp. 167–172.

YARCZOWER, M., and M. E. BITTERMAN, 1965. Stimulus generalizations in the goldfish. In *Stimulus Generalizations*. D. Mostofsky, ed. Stanford University Press, pp. 179–192.

16 Neural Information Processing with Stimulus Feature Extractors

GERHARD WERNER

ABSTRACT The complex stimulus properties to which certain classes of neurons are sensitive fall into two broad categories: One, consisting of movement or temporal modulation of stimuli; the other, representing stationary spatial patterns. The comparison between stimulus feature-sensitive neural mechanisms in the visual and the somesthetic system suggests that the stimulus features reflecting movement and change of stimuli play a role in directing the receptor sheet to positions relative to the stimulus object, which enable other feature detectors to respond to their appropriate stationary patterns. This conception emphasizes the serial aspect of information acquisition in perception: Each sample of stationary sense impressions would in this view be the result of neural activity in many sensory channels in parallel, and these samples would be acquired by movement of the receptor sheet into successive positions under guidance by neurons that signal stimulus motion and change. There is some evidence that this form of conjoint activity of motion and pattern-sensitive feature detectors would generate successions of sense impressions in a form suited for the encoding of spatial representations of stimulus objects.

Introduction

THE STUDY OF perception, like that of any other field of inquiry, starts from some observational facts and seeks explanations for them. The facts in perception are the way things appear to the naive observer. Hence, they are subjective and personal. In this, the subject matter of perception is unique among the sciences, for subjective experience is not publicly observable as the facts of science are generally required to be (Rock, 1970b).

In spite of this special status of the subject matter, the research methodology in perception is entirely comparable to that of other sciences. Once the conditions for a perceptual experience (for instance, the occurrence of a particular illusion) are established on which several observers agree, planned perturbations of the stimulus pattern can be employed as experimental tools. Stimuli that are randomly patterned in space (e.g., the familiar Rorschach test) or in time are among the most prolific procedures for this purpose. Such stimuli fulfill in the study of perception the role of the communication engineer's test signals that

GERHARD WERNER Department of Pharmacology, University of Pittsburgh, School of Medicine, Pittsburgh, Pennsylvania

reveal any bias in the information handling proclivities of a network (MacKay, 1965a). Furthermore, such stimuli may to some extent also permit the characterization of the information flow in the nervous system that must underlie the perceptual experience, and such stimuli enable the distinction between processes at the receptor level and in the central nervous system. The ingenious random dot stereograms of Julesz (1971) are a notable example of this approach.

An alternative approach starts from the experimentally established data of neurophysiology and attempts to examine the role that demonstrated neural events may play in perception. In this, we will encounter the three levels of discourse that MacKay (1965b) termed the *mind-talk*, the *brain-talk*, and the *computer-talk*: The language of self-observation is in this view irreducibly mentalistic, whereas the language of mechanistic description is appropriate only to the observer of another brain. The language and the ideas of the theory of information and control provide in this situation the right kind of hybrid status to serve as a conceptual bridge "enabling data gleaned in physiological terms to bear upon hypotheses in psychological terms, and *vice versa*" (MacKay, 1965b).

Beyond merely providing an *interlingua* for expressing relations between psychological and physiological phenomena (MacKay, 1967), the theory of information processing also promoted in recent years the emergence of a new paradigm in psychology (Neisser, 1972); theoretical terms such as *storage*, *retrieval*, *recoding*, and others as well, are now frequently applied conceptual aids. In this framework, perceptual activity is understood to encompass all processes beginning with the translation of stimulus energy on receptors, and leading to reports of experiences or responses to that stimulation, as well as memory persisting beyond the termination of the stimulation. Hence, sensation, perception, memory, and cognition are viewed as a continuum in the processing of sensory information, as the latter acts upon and is transformed by the nervous system (Haber, 1969). Moreover, from the moment the concept of information was introduced, it became impossible to consider in the study of perceptual processes isolated stimuli apart from others that, although physically absent, belonged together with the one present in the same class (Broadbent, 1971).

These general comments are intended to set the stage and delineate a framework for examining the role of feature-extracting neurons in perception. The central question is whether the functional characteristics of feature-extracting neurons, as a neural subsystem, correspond with those required by the antecedent psychological theory of perceptual information processing; and what aspects of perceptual functions would correspond to the neural system of feature extractors (see Fodor, 1968).

Perceptual phenomena suggestive of feature extraction

Starting with an accidental observation in a BBC studio lined with slotted wall paper, MacKay (1957, 1961) was led to discover (and, in some instances, rediscover) a wide range of effects with the perception of regular, spatially repetitive patterns. As explanation, MacKay suggested that the direction of a contour is signaled in the nervous system in a manner such that the presence of many contours with the same direction results, as it were, in a *directional satiation*; concomitantly, the perception of contours in the complementary direction would prevail.

Subsequently, many other perceptual phenomena were described that seemed amenable to similar interpretation. For instance, Blakemore and Campbell (1969) and Campbell and Maffei (1970) discovered that prolonged inspection of a grid elevates the detection threshold for grids with the same and similar orientation and spatial frequency. This rise of perceptual threshold was also accompanied by a reduction of the stimulus evoked cortical potentials (see Campbell, earlier in this part). Similarly, specific adaptation for the direction in which a grating of low spatial frequency moves across the visual field can also occur (Pantle and Sekuler, 1969).

These observations, as well as the evidence for differential color adaptation of orientation specific edge detectors (McCollough, 1965; Held and Shattuck, 1971) in human visual perception, lend considerable plausibility to the idea that the proximal stimulus on the retina is, at some stage in the visual information processing, decomposed into certain parts (or features); that these features engage independent information transmitting elements; and that these elements can be equated with the stimulus feature-sensitive neurons which had been demonstrated in the visual cortex of the cat (Hubel and Wiesel, 1962, 1965; Nikara et al., 1968; Campbell et al., 1968), monkey (Hubel and Wiesel, 1968) and man (Marg et al., 1968).

An intriguing observation by Richards (1971) adds an element of drastic realism to this conjecture: The visual displays that arise during ophthalmic migraines can have the appearance of serrated arcs illustrated in Figure 1,

whereby each line segment in the perceived display would be the perceptual counterpart of the neural discharges in a cluster of cortical cells for which the same line orientation is the trigger stimulus.

Lest we commit the "fallacy of early success," some

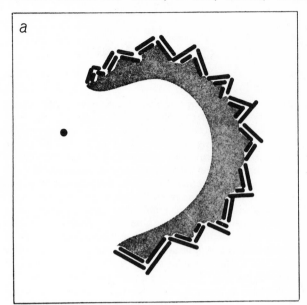

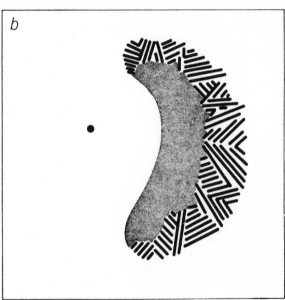

FIGURE 1 Fortification illusions of migraines, showing in (a) and (b) two appearances of their expanding boundaries. In the simplest type (a), the arc encircling a transient region of blindness (gray) is serrated and consists of two lines about as bright as an overhead fluorescent lamp; the lines oscillate in brightness at about 5 cycle/sec, with all the inside lines *on* when all the outside lines are *off*, and vice versa. In (b), a more complex appearance of a fortification illusion is shown. In each case, the gray area represents a transient region of blindness that moves outward from the point of fixation (black dot in figures), roughly parallel to the expanding arc. (From W. Richards, 1971.)

complicating issues need to be raised. Among these is the startling finding that colored aftereffects produced by parallel stripes or spirals may last for as long as six weeks (Stromeyer and Mansfield, 1970): It strains the neurophysiologist's imagination to assume that the activity of cortical feature-detecting neurons would, likewise, be affected throughout this period of time. Also, why does the adaptation to a certain orientation in a stimulus pattern produce as aftereffect a pattern with orthogonal orientation? Why did the adaptation not lead to a diffuse image, sparing only the adapted pattern, as is actually the case in audition? After exposure to auditory white noise from which a narrow frequency band is filtered out, the subjects report hearing a faint pitch at the center frequency of that filter (Zwicker, 1964). Thus, to account for the different adaptation response in the visual system, some special assumptions about interactions between feature-detecting neurons need to be introduced.

These unresolved issues barely detract from the elegance and conceptual simplicity of Sutherland's (1959, 1968) outline of a theory of visual pattern recognition. This theory anticipated and now rests, partly, on the well-known properties of feature-detecting neurons in the visual cortex (Hubel and Wiesel, 1962, 1965, 1968) that signal stimulus properties of different degrees of complexity. This complexity increases further with the projection from striate and prestriate cortex to the inferotemporal lobe (Gross et al., 1972). Two chief organizational principles seem to prevail: The first is the increase of receptive field size, leading with the inferotemporal neurons to the inclusion of the fovea into each neuron's receptive field; as a result, neurons signal the occurrence of their adequate stimulus with increasing independence from the actual site of stimulus impingement on the retina, as one progresses along the visual pathway. The second principle consists of increasing specificity of the adequate stimulus and, hence, progressive gain of information conveyed by a neural response (see Whitsel et al., 1972): The discharge of a neuron that responds to an edge in a particular orientation provided that edge ends at a certain point (hypercomplex cells of Hubel and Wiesel) is, informationally, much richer than is the discharge of a neuron that merely signals the presence of a light bar with a particular orientation (simple cells of Hubel and Wiesel). In somatic sensibility, a similar increase of complexity of stimulus features occurs: Some neurons in somatic sensory area 1 signal direction of stimulus motion over circumscript cutaneous receptive fields (Whitsel et al., 1972), whereas neurons in cytoarchitectural area 5 respond to more complex stimulus patterns, involving multiple joints and skin areas (Duffy and Burchfield, 1971).

Sutherland's outline of a theory also introduces the concept of an abstract description of the relation between the features signaled by these processing neural elements, which would take the form of an abstract symbolism, not unlike that of a formal language for processing and identifying pictorial structures by computers (Clowes, 1967, 1971); the relation of *join*, *next-to*, *inside*, *larger than*, etc., are examples of the presumed descriptive vocabulary.

According to this theory, when a shape is shone on the retina, it is analyzed into component parts by the feature-signaling neurons that function as the processor elements; memorizing or recognition of that shape requires then a recoding of the processor output according to some rules for description of pictures. This description is thought to be of sufficient generality that size, brightness, and position invariance of the perceived stimuli can be attained. The detailed logic of this process is expected to be so complex that a refinement of the theory, notably with the help of computer simulation, would have to precede any attempt to study its implementation in the nervous system.

The two components of Sutherland's proposal place an essential difference between available neurophysiological data and perceptual performance into clear focus: The former consist at present of descriptions of *local* properties of neural elements, or small groups of such elements, but the latter deals with the *global* aspects of perception. This difference prompts three questions that we will address in sequence: First, is the signaling of stimulus features by neurons as invariant and as independent of global stimulus properties as is often tacitly assumed? Second, what can be learned about the contribution of feature-detecting neurons to the global mechanisms of perception from the rules governing stimulus equivalence in transposition experiments? And, third, what place could feature-extracting neurons occupy in the acquisition of stimulus information and in perceptual learning?

Short-term changes of neural stimulus features

The observations of Horn and Hill (1969), Spinelli (1970), and Denney and Adarjani (1972) put the notion of immutability of visual stimulus feature detectors in doubt: In some neurons of the cat's visual cortex, the axis of an elongated receptive field appears to tilt concomitantly with head tilt, suggesting that the receptive field can maintain within limits its orientation in space, or at least undergo some less specific alteration with changes in excitation of vestibular statoreceptors (Schwartzkroin, 1972).

The observation by Hubel et al. (1959) that a class of neurons in the auditory cortex responds to acoustical stimuli only if the subject "pays attention" introduced the notion that the behavioral context in which a certain stimulus is applied determines its adequacy to elicit a neuronal response. The apparent significance of this modulation of neural responses by behavioral context is underscored by the finding of Miller et al. (1972) that the intensity of a neural response in macaques trained in an auditory discrimination task depends on whether or not the subjects are actually required to perform the learned response to the sensory cue. There is now also some accumulating evidence that the state of attention and vigilance can affect the sensitivity of neurons to stimulus features: Roppolo et al. (1972) have shown that neurons, which signal in the alert state the direction in which a cutaneous stimulus moves across the receptive field, may lose this directional specificity during periods of light sleep or drowsiness. However, it is not yet established whether more subtle behavioral contingencies, like the importance of a certain stimulus feature as cue in a behavioral task, can affect the specificity of the neural response to that same stimulus feature.

Morrell (1967) achieved a different type of modification of neural responses in studies that involved the repeated pairing of a trigger stimulus with a previously ineffective stimulus; eventually the latter stimulus becomes also effective in eliciting a neural response. Moreover, clusters of neurons were identified in parastriate cortex that responded to visual *and* auditory stimuli, provided the sound source was located in the neuron's receptive field for visual stimuli (Morrell, 1972). One might argue that such neurons are specific for events occurring at a certain locus in space and disregard the modality of the stimulus.

There is, finally, one more ambiguity in the signaling capability of feature-sensitive neurons: In the experimental studies, such neurons are conventionally classified according to their *best stimulus*, which is that stimulus configuration which elicits the maximal response; a less than maximal·response merely indicates departure from the optimal stimulus but not the direction of departure, nor does it indicate which component of the stimulus configuration was altered. Moreover, at least in one case, namely the class of neurons in primate somatic sensory area I, which signal directions of stimulus motion on the

skin, there appears an entire spectrum of *tuning*. These neurons differ widely in the range of orientations along which their responses differ with stimulus movement in opposing directions (Figure 2).

At least to some extent, these considerations tend to obscure the neatness of operational segregation into a class of stable processing elements on the one hand, and the hypothetical generator of an abstract description of the stimulus content; rather, it appears that the processing elements themselves would already be capable of performing some of the tasks required for insuring a stable perceptual world and for taking into account the context in which the stimulus occurs. In that sense, activity in *individual* stimulus feature detecting neurons hardly meets the requirements for a neural code of stimulus properties, although a *population* of such neurons may do so, albeit in a more complex manner that escapes experimental analysis with current methods (Perkel and Bullock, 1968).

Lessons from stimulus transposition

An interesting conceptualization of certain forms of perceptual constancies was proposed by Hoffman (1970); it rests on the generalization that neurons comprising certain cortical projection areas are not only arranged to topological maps of their respective receptor sheets but, in addition, are also sensitive and, therefore, represent in some sense particular local orientations and movement directions in the stimulus field. Hence, these cortical projection patterns may be viewed as vector fields, each stimulus orientation and direction singling out a set of neurons for which the particular orientation or direction is a "feature." Accordingly, stimulus contours and textures would be represented as appropriate alignments of orientation indicating field elements. Hoffman (1970) then proposed that certain basic invariances of perception, such as size or shape constancy, can be interpreted in terms of the operation of continuous transformation groups on the cortical representation of the field of view.

FIGURE 2 The contribution of a selected region of the receptive field to the cortical neuronal response as a function of the direction of stimulus motion. To generate each of the polar plots of this figure, the moving stimuli were applied at a variety of intersecting orientations within the receptive field, as is indicated in the accompanying figurine. The response profiles obtained of each stimulus orientation were arranged to permit identification of those *bins* that correspond to the point of chord intersection in the receptive field. The mean discharge rate per stimulus (expressed in impulse/sec) in these bins reflects the contribution of that portion of the receptive field to the neuronal response as the direction of brush advance is varied. Each direction of stimulus motion (identified by the direction of the arrow heads on the figurines) is assigned a number that corresponds to one of the heavy points on the circumference of the polar plots. The distance of these points from the origin of the coordinate system measures the neuronal response (in impulse/sec) generated by traversing the receptive field center in the direction identified by the appropriate number. Each stimulus was replicated 25 times. The circle around the origin of the coordinate system represents the level of spontaneous activity. The length of the interrupted radial line in each plot represents a calibration value of 50 impulse/sec/stimulus. (A) A "symmetrical" S-I neuron for the magnitude of neuronal response is independent of stimulus direction. (B, C, and D) "Asymmetric" S-I neurons that displayed direction selectivity at certain chord orientations. The stimulus velocities employed were 63 mm/sec (neuron A); 56 mm/sec (neuron B); 39 mm/sec (neuron C); and 236 mm/sec (neuron D). (From Whitsel et al., 1972, with the permission of the American Physiological Society.)

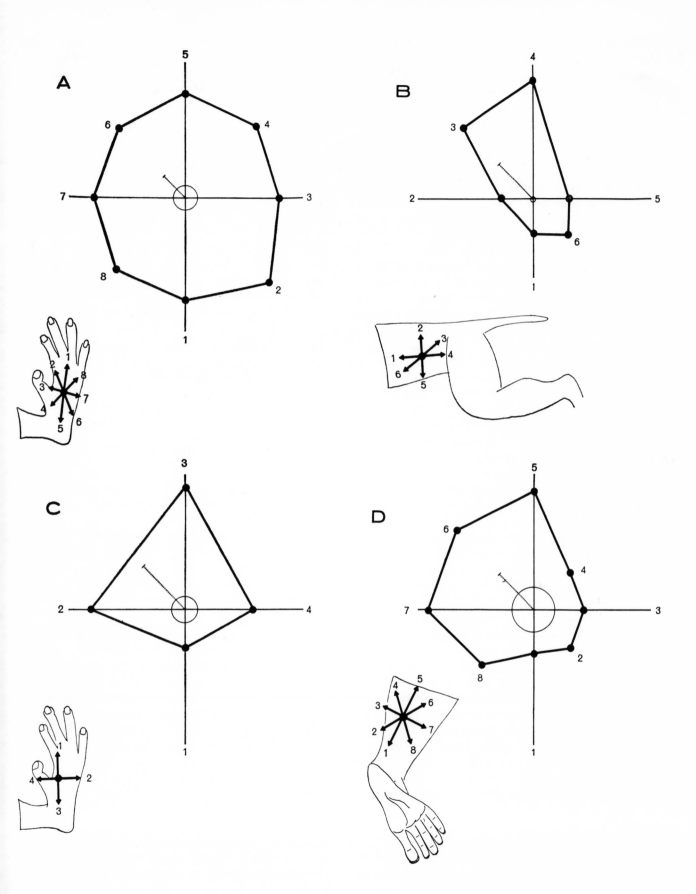

There are, however, limitations to the general applicability of this concept or, at least, situations in which additional factors come to play a role, for some stimulus transformations do not yield perceptual constancies, in spite of the fact that these stimulus transformations themselves possess group structure by virtue of the fact that each stimulus transformation has an inverse and that consecutive execution of transformations is again a transformation. One example is of stimulus discrimination when patterns are rotated. Recent work by Carlson (1972) with macaques, shown in Figure 3 illustrates that orientation plays a part in the definition of what we mean by the form or shape of an object (Hake, 1966).

This along with similar evidence from studies with subhuman primates suggests that the comparison of discriminanda transposed by rotation or reflection (mirror-image symmetry) is primarily based on some localized part of the figure; the site of the shape most significantly involved in the judgment of similarity or difference of the transposed shapes is, most often, the top or the bottom of the figures (Riopelle et al., 1969). This might also be related to the numerous observations with children, some of which date back to Ernst Mach (1886), that some kinds of rotations and reversals have more effect on transposition than others (for review, see Reese, 1968).

In short, patterns *can* be recognized despite rotation; but this accomplishment depends on rather complex mechanisms. The perceiver seems to construct within the figure an axis that defines some part as the top, and another as the bottom. Only then is he able to perform the comparison with another pattern previously presented. This circumstance precludes any simple account of the role of feature-sensitive neurons in pattern recognition and identification (see Neisser, 1966; Rock, 1970a). Moreover, Blakemore and Campbell (1969) have emphasized the difficulties that a feature-analyzing mechanism for spatial frequency—while accomplishing generalization for size most effectively—would encounter if it also had to generalize orientation.

Active processes in perception

There are two broad senses in which an organism has been said to be an *active perceiver* and perception to be an active process (Gyr et al., 1966). In the first sense, the perceiver's contribution consists of exploratory search of stimulation and variation in sensory input; activity in this sense involves movements of parts of the body (including the eyes) that lead to variations in the position of receptors relative to the stimuli. Thus, interaction between sensory and motor events becomes part of the information acquisition in perception. In the second sense, active perception stresses transactions between the observer and

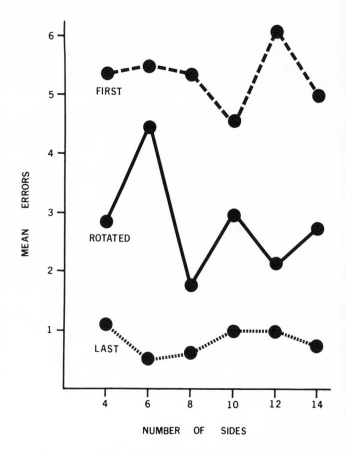

FIGURE 3 Monkeys were taught successive visual discriminations between pairs of random figures, both figures in a pair having the same number of sides. After criterion performance was achieved on each problem, the figures were rotated 180° and an additional 20 trials were given. The figure shows the mean errors as a function of the number of sides, on the first 20 trials of a problem (FIRST), the last 20 trials (LAST), and the subsequent 20 trials with the rotated figures (ROTATED). Errors after rotation were intermediate between and significantly different from errors on both the first and last 20 trials. This suggests that rotation only partially disrupts discrimination performance; subjects neither treated the rotated figures as comprising an entirely new problem, nor were they unaffected by the change in orientation. (From Carlson, 1972, with the permission of the Psychonomic Society.)

the environment to which the former may contribute a judgment-like activity (Helmholtz, 1867; Gregory, 1969), or memories from past experiences (Postman, 1955), or some form of "trial-and-check" process that leads to the structuring of percepts (Solley and Murphy, 1960; Miller et al., 1960).

Clearly, these two aspects of active perception are in no way mutually exclusive, for its appears plausible that past experiences can provide the strategies for employing sensory-motor mechanisms in the service of acquisition of stimulus information. To sharpen the issue, we should contrast this with sensory inputs simply impinging as a result of accidental orientation of sense organs, or with inputs provided by some outside source, such as the experimenter.

What role can we attribute to stimulus feature signaling neurons in this complex information transaction between an observer, who has become familiar with certain redundancies and regularities in his environment, and changing patterns of stimulus energy?

Vision and movement

Broadly speaking, the past decade has led to the emergence of the principle of *separability of pattern and place* (Horridge, 1968) in the ways in which visual information is processed in the nervous system. One line of evidence for this comes from complete lesions of the striate cortex in monkeys. Such lesions produce deficits in object recognition and pattern discrimination but leave detection and localization of stationary and moving visual stimuli, as well as visually guided movements in relation to those stimuli, intact (Humphrey, 1970). This residual capacity implies at least some form of figure-ground differentiation within the sensory field; yet, this field remains perceptually unstructured, because forms are not recognized. Hence, Humphrey's (1970) imaginative proposal that spatial information comes in this case indirectly: Eye movements would be guided by the sensory field, and there would be a tendency automatically to fixate visually differentiated figures; the cortically deprived monkey, thus, knows of the location of an object by monitoring, internally, where her eyes are looking. In effect, the monkey has learned to "use her hands as an extension of her eyes; in a real sense she sees *with*, not through, the eye" (Humphrey, 1970).

The second source of evidence is that each hemisphere can function independently of the other in pattern identification and discrimination when the commissural connections between the two cortices are cut; thus, a stimulus identification learned through one eye can no longer be performed when the same stimulus is presented to the other eye, as is the case with intact commissural connection (Trevarthen, 1967).

The conclusions from these and similar studies point to an anatomical differentiation between two neural systems with different competence for processing visual information: One, involved in locating and orienting toward targets in the visual field, which is not affected by severance of hemispheric connections and, thus, composed of retinomesencephalic projections; the other involving retinotelencephalic projections capable of processing visual information of patterns and shapes (Schneider, 1967, 1969).

Does stimulus feature detection in the retinostriate and in the mesencephalic system differ in a manner that could account for their different role in visual perception?

The cellular stratification of the superior colliculi is suggestive of a hierarchy of neural functions within them: In the macaque, the large majority of neurons in the upper layers respond to small stationary spots of light though their receptive fields are large, and they are strongly excited by movement of a light spot in any direction within the receptive field; but they are not affected by shape, size, or orientation of a stimulus. In addition, there is emphasis on novel stimuli, because responses decline with repeated stimulus application (Humphrey 1968). Thus, local change is the *one* aspect about a stimulus that these neurons signal. A more specific operation is carried out by a minority of neurons in this layer because they respond only to certain directions of stimulus motion and not to others (Wurtz and Goldberg, 1972).

Finally, there are neurons that discharge with increased vigor whenever a visual stimulus becomes the target of an eye movement: Some are related to saccadic eye movements, and others, notably in the intermediate gray layers, fire just prior to an eye movement made to fixate a particular area of the visual field. Each of these latter neurons has a certain direction of eye movement associated with its most intense discharge, which is independent of the absolute position of the eye, either prior to or at the end point of the movement. Some of these neurons also have visual receptive fields that, before movement, correspond roughly to the spatial position to which the eye is directed by the neuron's discharge (Wurtz and Goldberg, 1972).

In its entirety, this neuronal assembly consistently filters change and novelty in the visual field as "parcels of information" (Lettvin and Maturana; see Ploog, 1971), which lead to the issuing of specific commands. Whether these commands are related to the mechanism of foveation (i.e., target acquisition by saccades and target maintenance by smooth pursuit) (Schiller and Koerner, 1971), or whether they signal to other regions of the brain that an eye movement is impending (i.e., a corollary discharge; Sperry, 1950; Teuber, 1960) is still uncertain. In any case, however, there is a clear difference between the nature of the events in the visual field that affect the neurons of the superior colliculi and the stimuli for which a substantial contingent of neurons in the striate cortex is *tuned*. The emphasis of these latter neurons is on the spatial layout of contours, present in *stationary* patterns in the visual field (Wurtz, 1969; Noda et al., 1971).

Although so clearly distinct in neuronal response characteristics, there is strong support for the concept that cortex and midbrain (i.e., superior colliculi and pretectum) jointly contribute to the learning of visual pattern discrimination tasks. Anatomical evidence establishes the existence of ascending tectal pathways, supplied mostly from the peripheral retina (Wilson and Toyne, 1970), to certain parts of visual cortex via posterior thalamic nuclei (Diamond and Hall, 1969; Graybiel, Part 3 of this volume); and the behavioral studies of Berlucchi et al. (1972) demonstrated the essential role of superior colliculi and pretectum in the acquisition of visual discrimination performance. It appears that visual cortical areas (notably circumstriate cortex) have come into possession of the best of two worlds: The stimulus motion detection in the peripheral retina as source of eye movement commands, and the stationary contour coding in the foveal component of the geniculostriate system. Does this juxtaposition of extrafoveal, eye-movement related and foveal, pattern sensitive cortex in the circumstriate belt contain a clue for its role in pattern vision?

Familiar visual scenes can be recognized if presented in a brief flash, too short to enable scanning by eye movements. However, when eye movements are permitted to occur, and when they are required for the perception of a novel stimulus pattern, they externalize, as it were, the information processing in the visual system (Yarbus, 1967; Jeannerod et al., 1968). An extreme position in this line of thought is taken in the *scan path theory* of Noton (1970; see also, Noton and Stark, 1971), which proposes that the central representation of a visual pattern consists of a sequence of sensory and motor memory traces, recording individual features of the pattern and the eye movements required to pass from feature to feature across the pattern. More generally, and in keeping with the ability for tachistoscopic perception of familiar visual scenes, is the alternative suggestion that entire samples of visual scenes would be acquired at each eye position. Each individual sample would in this view be the result of information processing in many visual channels in parallel, and these samples would be acquired by successive eye fixations.

The question is, could the visual cortex (notably the circumstriate area) implement the acquisition of sequencies of "snapshots" of the visual scene by bringing one image sample after the other into foveal vision? It could accomplish this in some sense automatically, at least on first presentation of a novel pattern when no prior strategies for inspection are available from past experience. As an eye movement brings a new visual scene into foveal "focus," other components of the visual field would activate neurons in the peripheral retina; their activity would generate in the colliculo-pulvinar-extrastriate system the "program" for the next eye movement, and so on. Between eye movements, the geniculostriate projec-

tion system could apply its "static" feature analyzing operation *seriatim* to one sample from the visual scene after the other.

In some sense, we have made a full circle: While "separability of pattern and place" was suggested by the differences in the central routing of feature signals for structural (i.e., purely spatial) and for time-space dependent (i.e., motion) aspects of the stimulus, we have come to see ways in which the neural responses to these two classes of visual stimuli can jointly constitute a *description* of a stimulus pattern. This description has some formal analogy to the requirements that were found to suffice for mimicking certain forms of perceptual and cognitive functions in artificial intelligence studies (Simon and Newell, 1971). The analogy consists of (a) serial information processing and (b) the individual data items being "linked" to lists (in an abstract sense) in which the sequential eye movement commands are the "pointers" marking the order in which the list is structured.

The tactile apprehension of object quality and shape

Identification of objects by palpation is based on the concurrent sensory influx from cutaneous touch and articular position and motion. Palpation encompasses at least two distinct activities: One, consisting of the shaping of the hand for grasping the object, or parts of it; the other consisting of displacing the hand by successive movements along the object's contours and surfaces.

As one would expect, the manipulation plays a major role as the observer seems to be trying to obtain mechanical events at the skin in various combinations and at various places. Gibson (1962) quantitated the superiority of "active" over "passive" touch: Shapes were to be identified when they were either pressed into the palm of the hand or accessible to exploration by the finger tips. The result was highly impressive, for in passive touch, correct matches were only half as often attained as in active touch.

Neurophysiological and neuroanatomical investigation characterized in recent years the neural system that evolution specialized for active touch. The evidence comes from the currently ongoing reassessment of the role of the dorsal column, medial lemniscal pathway and its cortical projection in somesthesis. It has been known for some time that lesions of somatic sensory area I (S-I) in the monkey impair shape discrimination by palpatory exploration of the stimulus object (Orbach and Chow, 1959); yet, tactile thresholds are not altered (Schwartzman and Semmes, 1971). Furthermore, lesions of area 5 in the parietal lobe that receives a heavy projection from S-I (Jones and Powell, 1969) also affect active tactual discrimination selectively (Ettlinger et al., 1966). In contrast, discrimination of passively received cutaneous stimuli involves primarily the second somatic sensory area (Glassman, 1970; Schwartzman and Semmes, 1971).

As regards the dorsal columns themselves, evidence has accumulated that they are indispensable for the execution of tasks in which accurate timing and sequencing of limb projections into extracorporeal space are important aspects (Dubrovsky et al., 1971; Melzack and Bridges, 1971). Earlier, Gilman and Denny-Brown (1966) concluded that the dorsal columns constitute an essential part of the neural mechanisms for projected limb movement into ambient space and, in particular, for the fine contactual orienting reactions of forelimbs. In contrast, there are numerous studies of tactile discrimination tasks with passively applied cutaneous stimuli that do not attribute more than, at best, a secondary role to the dorsal columns (for review, see Semmes, 1972).

Therefore, Semmes (1969) and Wall (1970) can muster strong support for their contention that sensory information in the dorsal column pathway and its principal cortical receiving area in S-I is available in a form that is primarily suited for guiding object manipulation and exploration by the limbs. In this conception, the dorsal columns function essentially as an alerting system, setting into motion mechanisms for analyzing sensory information arriving through parallel channels and directing motor search for additional data. The cutaneous afferents from the *distal* limbs receive in this a preferential treatment, for they reach their destination in S-I almost exclusively *via* the dorsal columns, while afferents from more proximal portions of the limbs and from the trunk ascend also in the dorsolateral tract of the spinal cord: Thus, the cortical projection fields of the distal portions of hand and feet appear, essentially, as islands of dorsal column projection within S-I (Dreyer et al., 1973).

Is this an analogy to the juxtaposition of foveal and extrafoveal representations in the visual cortex, separating also in the somesthetic system movement detection from pattern analysis? The answer is incomplete, but as far as it is available, it supports at least the expectation of movement signaling neurons in somesthetic cortex: It has recently been possible to identify in S-I a class of neurons that single out certain orientations of chords in their cutaneous receptive fields for which responses to stimuli moving in opposite directions differ substantially. Direction and orientation of stimulus motion on the skin assume, thereby, the character of a stimulus feature (Whitsel et al., 1972). Figure 4 illustrates that the orientational and directional specificity of these neurons increases, as a rule, at higher stimulus velocities and

reaches an optimum in the range of 100–200 mm/sec. This is also the velocity range for the best texture identification of objects moving over the skin of humans (Katz, 1925).

Adherence to the prototype of the visual system would suggest that these directionally selective detectors for stimulus movement on the skin surface play a role for triggering manual grasping automatisms. In both cases a moving stimulus would direct a receptor sheet to "capture" the stimulus. However, much of somesthesis, being a phylogenetic latecomer, introduces an intriguing difference. As far as is known, there are no mesencephalic centers for dynamic stimulus features in somesthesis, which would be comparable to tectum and superior colliculi in vision, or inferior colliculi in audition. Instead, movement related stimulus features appear to any appreciable extent for the first time as far rostral in the projection path as S-I, exclusively as a result of intracortical information processing (Whitsel et al., 1972). It may be safe to predict that movement related features occur in greater diversity and specificity in cortical areas beyond S-I.

Of the various forms of grasping automatisms (Seyffarth and Denny-Brown, 1948), the *instinctive grasp reaction* appears as a promising candidate upon which voluntary prehension and palpatory exploration of the objects of touch could build (see Twitchell, 1965): The moving contact stimulus to any part of the hand elicits a highly integrated response that places the hand in a position of readiness for a series of light palpating and groping movements and is eventually followed by a final grasping of the object. The conjecture is that such automatisms are the building blocks of haptic sensibility.

The unity of the phenomenal object in perception

The preceding sections assembled some of the arguments in favor of the general concept that different classes of neurons "attend" to different aspects of a stimulus. Some of the stimulus features reflect movement and change of the stimulus and appear to take part in directing the receptor sheet to positions relative to the stimulus, which enable other feature detectors to register glimpses of stationary patterns. This conception emphasizes the *serial* aspect of information acquisition in perception.

In an imaginative experiment that consisted of moving objects or patterns behind a hole whose diameter was such that at most one corner could be seen at the time, Hochberg (1968) proved at least for vision that the serial presentation of sequential views of a shape was *sufficient* for its identification. However, this experiment also underscores the complexity of the further processing of

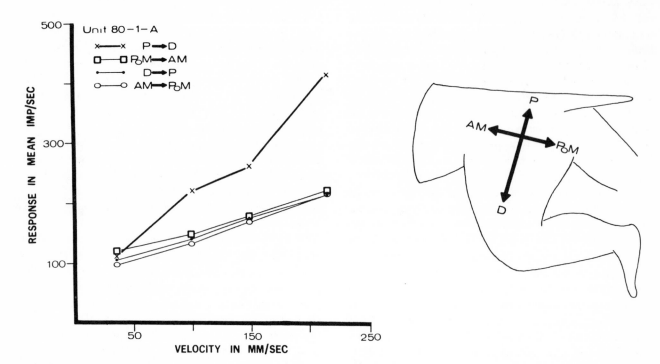

FIGURE 4 Contribution of a selected region of the receptive field to cortical neuronal response as a function of velocity and direction of stimulus motion. To obtain these plots, the response profiles resulting from 25 replications of each of the four directions of stimulus motion were arranged to permit identification of those bins that correspond to the point of chord intersection in the receptive field. The mean discharge rate per stimulus (expressed in impulses per second) in these bins is plotted against velocity. The velocity dependence of the response at the point of chord intersection varies dramatically with the direction of stimulus motion; i.e., a preferred direction of the stimulus motion became increasingly predominant (namely, the P → D direction) at the higher stimulus velocities. AM, anterior midline; PoM, posterior midline; P, proximal; D, distal. (From Whitsel et al., 1972, with the permission of the American Physiological Society.)

the serially obtained views that must be assumed. There must be perceptual memory for retaining the sequential views in some short-term memory and some recoding to larger "perceptual units" (see Neisser, 1966). These later stages of information processing are accessible to identification and characterization by perceptual masking and figural aftereffects (Haber, 1969).

Upon entering these stages of information processing, differences between sense modalities play a rapidly diminishing role (Massaro, 1972), except for a clear distinction in the handling of spatial as opposed to verbal information (Brooks, 1968). This enables the trading of spatial information acquired by different sense modalities

in, at least, two forms: First, sense information acquired in one modality can become organized in the spatial schema of another modality; an example of this is the preference for representing spatial location and shapes in visual terms, even when based on tactile input (Scholtz, 1957; Attneave and Benson, 1969). Second, man and some subhuman primates (Davenport and Rogers, 1970) become capable of crossmodal comparisons of shapes. But, although freed from constraints by sense modalities, this supramodal mechanism is still sensitive to the manner of stimulus presentation: It only operates effectively if the patterns are presented in spatiotemporal succession, for instance by describing them with a stylus as paths in space and time (Krauthamer, 1968). Hence, this perceptual coding mechanism requires for its optimal effectiveness that stimulus patterns be presented as successions of sense impressions.

This circumstance puts the function of the motion and pattern sensitive neural elements and pathways into a new light: For, according to the conception presented earlier, their conjoint activity would generate sense information in just the form that matches the information handling proclivity of the coding system for spatial representation.

REFERENCES

ATTNEAVE, F., and B. BENSON, 1969. Spatial coding of tactual stimulation. *J. Expl. Psychol.* 81:216–222.

BERLUCCHI, G., J. M. SPRAGUE, J. LEVY, and A. C. DiBERARDINO, 1972. Protection and superior colliculus in visually guided behavior and in flux and form discrimination in the cat. *J. Comp. Physiol. Psychol.*, Monogr. 75, No. 1, p. 123–172.

BLAKEMORE, C., and F. W. CAMPBELL, 1969. On the existence of neurons in the human visual system selectively sensitive to the orientation and size of retinal images. *J. Physiol.* (*London*) 203:237–260.

BROADBENT, D. E., 1971. *Decision and Stress.* New York: Academic Press.

BROOKS, L. R., 1968. Spatial and verbal components of the act of recall. *Canad. J. Psychol./Rev. Canad. Psychol.* 22:349–368.

CAMPBELL, F. W., B. G. CLELAND, G. F. COOPER, and C. ENROTH-CUGELL, 1968. The angular selectivity of visual cortical cells to moving gratings. *J. Physiol.* (*London*) 198:237–250.

CAMPBELL, F. W., and L. MAFFEI, 1970. Electrophysiological evidence for the existence of orientation and size detectors in the human visual system. *J. Physiol.* (*London*) 207:635–652.

CARLSON, K. R., 1973. Visual discrimination of random figures by rhesus monkeys. *Anim. Learn. Behav.* 1:23–35.

CLOWES, M. B., 1967. Perception, picture processing and computers. In *Machine Intelligence*, 1:181–197. N. L. Collins and D. Michie, eds. New York: Elsevier Publishing Company.

CLOWES, M. B., 1971. On seeing things. *Artif. Intell.* 2:79–116.

DAVENPORT, R. K., and C. M. ROGERS, 1970. Intermodal equivalence of stimuli in apes. *Science* 168:279–280.

DENNEY, D., and C. ADARJANI, 1972. Orientation specificity of visual cortical neurons after head tilt. *Exp. Brain Res.* 14:312–317.

DIAMOND, I. T., and W. C. HALL, 1969. Evolution of neocortex. *Science* 164:251–262.

DREYER, D. A., R. SCHNEIDER, C. METZ, and B. L. WHITSEL, 1973. Differential contributions of spinal pathways to the body representation in the postcentral gyrus. *J. Neurophysiol.* (in press).

DUBROVSKY, B., E. DAVELAAR, and E. GARCIA-RILL, 1971. The role of dorsal columns in serial order acts. *Expl. Neurol.* 33:93–102.

DUFFY, F. H., and J. L. BURCHFIELD, 1971. Somatosensory system-organizational hierarchy from single units in monkey area 5. *Science* 172:273–275.

ETTLINGER, G., H. B. MORTON, and A. MOFFETT, 1966. Tactile

discrimination performance in the monkey: The effect of bilateral posterior parietal and lateral frontal ablations, and of callosal section. *Cortex* 2:6–29.

FODOR, J. A., 1968. *Psychological Explanation: An introduction to the Philosophy of Psychology.* New York: Random House.

GIBSON, J. J., 1962. Observations on active touch. *Psychol. Rev.* 69:477–491.

GILMAN, S., and D. DENNY-BROWN, 1966. Disorders of movement and behavior following dorsal column lesions. *Brain* 89:397–418.

GLASSMAN, R., 1970. Cutaneous discrimination and motor control following somatosensory cortical ablations. *Physiol. Behav.* 5:1009–1019.

GREGORY, R. L., 1969. On how so little information controls so much behavior. In *Towards a Theoretical Biology*, (an IBUS Symposium) Vol. 2, C. H. Waddington, ed. Chicago: Aldine Publishing Company, pp. 236–247.

GROSS, C. G., C. E. ROCHA-MIRANDA, and D. B. BENDER, 1972. Visual properties of neurons in inferotemporal cortex of macaque. *J. Neurophysiol.* 35:96-111.

GYR, J. W., J. S. BROWN, R. WILLEY, and A. ZIVIAN, 1966. Computer simulation and psychological theories of perception. *Psychol. Bull.* 65:174–192.

HABER, R. N., 1969. Introduction. In *Information-Processing Approaches to Visual Perception.* New York: Holt, Rinehart and Winston.

HAKE, H. W., 1966. Form discrimination and the invariance of form. In *Pattern Recognition*, L. Uhr, ed. New York: John Wiley & Sons, pp. 142–173.

HELD, R., and S. R. SHATTUCK, 1971. Color- and edge-sensitive channels in the human visual system: Tuning for orientation. *Science* 174:317–316.

HELMHOLTZ, H., 1867. *Handbuch der Physiologischen Optik.* Leipzig: Voss.

HIRSCH, H. V. B., 1972. Visual perception in cats after environmental surgery. *Exp. Brain Res.* 15:405–423.

HOCHBERG, JULIAN, 1968. In the mind's eye. In *Contemporary Theory and Research in Visual Perception*, R. N. Haber, ed. New York: Holt, Rinehart and Winston, pp. 309–331.

HOFFMAN, W. C., 1970. Higher visual perception as prolongation of the basic lie transformation group. *Math. Biosci.* 6:437–471.

HORN, J., and R. M. HILL, 1969. Modification of receptive fields of cells in the visual cortex occurring spontaneously and associated with bodily tilt. *Nature* (*London*) 221:186–188.

HORRIDGE, G. A., 1968. *Interneurons.* San Francisco: W. H. Freeman and Company.

HUBEL, D. H., C. O. HENSON, A. RUPPERT, and R. GALAMBOS, 1959. Attention units in the auditory cortex. *Science* 129:1279–1280.

HUBEL, D. H., and T. N. WIESEL, 1962. Receptive fields, binocular interaction and functional architecture in the cat's visual cortex. *J. Physiol.* (*London*) 160:106–154.

HUBEL, H., and T. N. WIESEL, 1965. Receptive fields and functional architecture in two non-striate visual areas (18 and 19) of the cat. *J. Neurophysiol.* 28:229–289.

HUBEL, D. H., and T. N. WIESEL, 1968. Receptive fields and functional architecture of monkey striate cortex. *J. Physiol.* (*London*) 195:215–243.

HUMPHREY, N. K., 1968. Responses to visual stimuli of units in the superior colliculus of rats and monkeys. *Exp. Neurol.* 20:312–340.

HUMPHREY, N. K., 1970. What the frog's eye tells the monkey's brain. *Brain, Behav., Evolut.* 3:324–337.

JEANNEROD, M., P. GERIN, and J. PERNIER, 1968. Deplacements et fixation du regard dans l'exploration libre d'une scène visuelle. *Vision Res.* 8:81–97.

JONES, E. G., and T. P. S. POWELL, 1969. Connexions of the somatic sensory cortex of the rhesus monkey. I. Ipsilateral cortical connexions. *Brain* 92:477–502.

JULESZ, B., 1971. *Foundations of Cyclopean Perception.* University of Chicago Press.

KATZ, D., 1925. Der Anfbau der Tast welt. Leipzig: Barth.

KRAUTHAMER, G., 1968. Form perception across sensory modalities. *Neuropsychologia* 6:105–113.

McCOLLOUGH, C., 1965. Color adaptation of edge-detectors in the human visual system. *Science* 149:1115–1116.

MACH, E., 1907. *The Analysis of Sensations and the Relation of the Psychical.* (Translated by C. M. Williams from the 1st ed. of *Die Analyse der Empfindungen und das Verhaltnis des Psychischen zum Physischen,* 1914). La Salle, Ill.: Open Court Publishing Company.

MACKAY, D. M., 1957. Moving visual images produced by regular spatial patterns. *Nature (London)* 180:849–850.

MACKAY, D. M., 1961. Interactive processes in visual perception. In *Sensory Communication,* W. A. Rosenblith, ed. Cambridge, Mass.: The MIT Press and John Wiley & Sons, pp. 339–355.

MACKAY, D. M., 1965a. Visual noise as a tool of research. *J. Gen. Psychol.* 72:181–197.

MACKAY, D. M., 1965b. A mind's eye view of the brain. In *Cybernetics of the Nervous System,* Progress in Brain Research, Vol. 17. N. Wiener and J. P. Schade, eds. New York: Elsevier Publishing Company, pp. 321–332.

MACKAY, D. M., 1967. Report on the symposium on neural communication. *IBRO Bull.* 6:5–18.

MARG, E., J. E. ADAMS, and B. RUTKIN, 1968. Receptive fields of cells in the human visual cortex. *Experientia* 24:348–350.

MASSARO, D. W., 1972. Prepreceptual images, processing time, and perceptual units in auditory perception. *Psychol. Rev.* 79:124–145.

MELZACK, R., and J. A. BRIDGES, 1971. Dorsal column contribution to motor behavior. *Exp. Neurol.* 33:53–68.

MILLER, G. A., E. GALANTER, and K. H. PRIBRAM, 1960. *Plans and the Structure of Behavior.* New York: Holt, Rinehart and Winston.

MILLER, J. M., D. SUTTON, B. PFINGST, A. RYAN, and R. BEATON, 1972. Single cell activity in the auditory cortex of Rhesus monkeys: Behavioral dependency. *Science* 177:449–451.

MORRELL, F., 1967. Electrical signs of sensory coding. In *The Neurosciences,* a Study Program. G. C. Quarton, T. Melnechuk, and F. O. Schmitt, eds. New York: The Rockefeller University Press.

MORRELL, F., 1972. Integrative properties of parastriate neurons. In *Brain and Human Behavior,* A. G. Karczmar, and J. C. Eccles, eds. New York: Springer-Verlag, pp. 259–289.

NEISSER, U., 1966. *Cognitive Psychology.* New York: Appleton-Century-Crofts.

NEISSER, U., 1972. A paradigm shift in psychology (Book review). *Science* 176:628–630.

NIKARA, T., P. O. BISHOP, and J. D. PETTIGREW, 1968. Analysis of retinal correspondence by studying receptive fields of binocular single units in cat striate cortex. *Exp. Brain Res.* 6:353–372.

NODA, H., R. B. FREEMAN, JR., B. GIES, and O. D. CREUTZFELDT, 1971. Neuronal responses in the visual cortex of awake cats to stationary and moving targets. *Exp. Brain Res.* 12:389–405.

NOTON, D., 1970. A theory of visual pattern perception. *IEEE Trans. Syst. Sci. Cybern.* 6:349–357.

NOTON, D., and L. STARK, 1971. Scanpaths in saccadic eye movements while viewing and recognizing patterns. *Vision Res.* 11:929–942.

ORBACH, J., and K. CHOW, 1959. Differential effects of resections of somatic areas I and II in monkeys. *J. Neurophysiol.* 22:195–203.

PANTLE, A., and R. SEKULER, 1969. Contrast response of human visual mechanisms sensitive to orientation and direction of motion. *Vision Res.* 9:397–406.

PERKEL, D. H., and T. H. BULLOCK, 1968. Neural coding. *Neurosciences Research Program Bulletin* 6(3).

PLOOG, D., 1971. The relevance of natural stimulus patterns for sensory information processes, *Brain Res.* 31:353–359.

POSTMAN, L., 1955. Association theory and perceptual learning. *Psychol. Rev.* 62:438–446.

REESE, H., 1968. *The Perception of Stimulus Relations.* New York: Academic Press.

RICHARDS, W., 1971. The fortification illusions of migraines. *Sci. Amer.* 224(5):88–96.

RIOPELLE, A. J., U. RAHM, N. ITOIGAWA, and W. A. DRAPER, 1964. Discrimination of mirror-image patterns by rhesus monkeys. *Percept. Motor Skills* 19:383–389.

ROCK, I., 1970a. Perception from the standpoint of psychology. *Res. Publ. Ass. Res. Nerv. Ment. Dis.* 48:139–149.

ROCK, I., 1970b. Toward a cognitive theory of perceptual constancy. In *Contemporary Scientific Psychology,* A. R. Gilgen, ed. New York: Academic Press.

ROPPOLO, J. R., D. DREYER, B. WHITSEL, and G. WERNER. Phencyclidine action on neural mechanism of somesthesis. *Neuropharmacology* (in press).

SCHILLER, P. H., and F. KOERNER, 1971. Discharge characteristics of single units in superior colliculus of the alert rhesus monkey. *J. Neurophysiol.* 34:920–936.

SCHNEIDER, G., 1967. Contrasting visuomotor functions of tectum and cortex in the golden hamster. *Psychol. Forsch.* 31:52–62.

SCHNEIDER, G. E., 1969. Two visual systems. *Science* 163:895–902.

SCHOLTZ, D. A., 1957. Die Grundsatze der Gestaltwahruehmung in der Haptik. *Acta Psychologica (Amst.)* 13:299–333.

SCHWARTZKROIN, P. A., 1972. The effect of body tilt on the directionality of units in cat visual cortex. *Exp. Neurol.* 36:498–506.

SCHWARTZMAN, R. J., and J. SEMMES, 1971. The sensory cortex and tactile sensitivity. *Expl. Neurol.* 33:147–158.

SEMMES, J., 1969. Protopathic and epicritic sensation: A reappraisal. In *Contribution to Clinical Neuropsychology.* A. L. Benton, ed. Chicago: Aldine Publishing Company, pp. 142–169.

SEMMES, J., 1972. Somesthetic effects of damage to the central nervous system. In *Handbook of Sensory Physiology,* A. Iggo, ed. Berlin: Springer-Verlag.

SEYFFARTH, H., and D. DENNY-BROWN, 1948. The grasp reflex and the instinctive grasp reaction. *Brain* 71(2):9–183.

SIMON, H. A., and A. NEWELL, 1971. Human problem solving: The state of the theory in 1970. *Amer. Psychol.* 26:145–159.

SOLLEY, C. M., and G. M. MURPHY, 1960. *Development of the Perceptual World.* New York: Basic Books.

SPERRY, R. W., 1950. Neural basis of the spontaneous optokinetic response produced by visual inversion. *J. Comp. Physiol. Psychol.* 43:482–489.

SPINELLI, D. N., 1970. Recognition of visual patterns. *Res. Publ. Ass. Res. Nerv. Ment. Dis.* 48:139–149.

STROMEYER, III, C. F., and R. J. W. MANSFIELD, 1970. Colored aftereffects produced with moving edges. *Perception and Psychophysics* 7:108–114.

SUTHERLAND, N. S., 1959. Stimulus analyzing mechanisms. *Proc. Symp. on Mechanization of Thought Processes*, Vol. 2, p. 575–609. London: H.M. Stationery Office.

SUTHERLAND, N. S., 1968. Outlines of a theory of visual pattern recognition in animals and man. *Proc. Roy. Soc. (Biol.)* 171: 297–317.

TEUBER, H., 1960. Perception. In *Handbook of Physiology*, Vol. 3, Section 1, J. Field, ed. Washington, D.C.: American Physiological Society, pp. 1595–1668.

TREVARTHEN, C. B., 1967. Two mechanisms of vision in primates. *Psychol. Forsch.* 31:299–337.

TREVARTHEN, C. B., 1970. Experimental evidence for a brain stem contribution to visual perception in man. *Brain, Behav., Evol.* 3:338–352.

TWITCHELL, T. E., 1965. The automatic grasping responses of infants. *Neuropsychologia* 3:247–259.

WALL, P. D., 1970. The sensory and motor role of impulses traveling in the dorsal columns towards cerebral cortex. *Brain* 93:505–524.

WERNER, G., B. L. WHITSEL, and L. M. PETRUCELLI, 1972. Data structure and algorithms in the primate somatosensory cortex. In *Brain and Human Behavior*, A. G. Karczmar, and J. C. Eccles, eds. Berlin: Springer-Verlag, pp. 164–186.

WHITSEL, B. L., J. R. ROPPOLO, and G. WERNER, 1972. Cortical information processing of stimulus motion on primate skin. *J. Neurophysiol.* 35:691–717.

WILSON, M. E., and M. J. TOYNE, 1970. Retino-tectal and corticotectal projection in *Macaca Mulatta. Brain Res.* 24: 395–406.

WURTZ, R. H., 1969. Visual receptive fields of striate cortex neurons in awake monkeys. *J. Neurophysiol.* 37:727–741.

WURTZ, H., and M. E. GOLDBERG, 1972. The role of the superior colliculus in visually evoked eye movements. In *Cerebral Control of Eye Movements and Motion Perception*, J. Dichgans and E. Bizzi, eds. Basel: Karger pp. 149–158.

YARBUS, A. L., 1967. *Eye Movements and Vision*. New York: Plenum Press.

ZWICKER, E., 1964. Negative afterimage in hearing. *J. Acoust. Soc. Amer.* 46:805–811.